Basics of

HUMAN ANATOMY

FOR

STUDENTS OF MEDICAL & ALLIED HEALTH SCIENCES

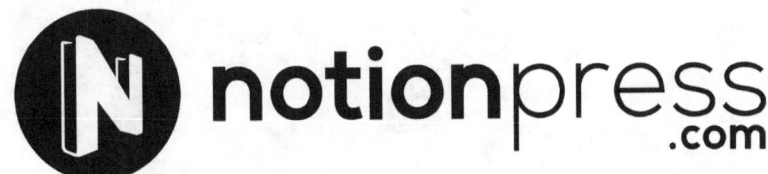

Basics of
HUMAN ANATOMY
— FOR —
STUDENTS OF MEDICAL & ALLIED HEALTH SCIENCES

General Anatomy and General Histology – Vol. 1

Dr. Najma Mobin

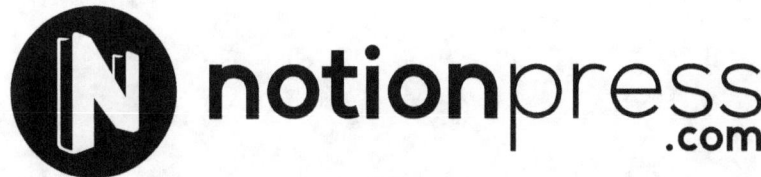

Notion Press

Old No. 38, New No. 6
McNichols Road, Chetpet
Chennai - 600 031

First Published by Notion Press 2017
Copyright © Dr. Najma Mobin 2017
All Rights Reserved.

ISBN 978-1-948473-05-7

Dedication

In the name of GOD the Most Gracious and Most Merciful.

I dedicate this book to my beloved parents:

Mr. Syed Jaffer Peer

&

Mrs. Syeda Badrunnisa

I thank my beloved husband **Mr. Mohammed Mobin** for his constant support and encouragement.

I thank my sweetest daughter **Ayesha Mobin Fathima** for being supportive.

I thank my dear brothers **Mr. Syed Ansar Peer** and **Mr. Syed Kausar Peer** for giving me confidence and being there with me as my supporting pillars all the time.

CONTENTS

FOREWORD

The basics of general anatomy and general histology are very essential to understand the human anatomy. The presentation of different topics is excellent with understandable explanations and relevant references to clinical aspects with a view to simplify and provide concise knowledge so that the students of all health science can derive maximum benefits.

It is a conventional handbook for histology which provides microscopic diagrams of H & E stained slides as well as hand drawn diagrams which helps the students for preparation and quick revision before the examination. The list of questions and MCQ's at the end of each chapter helps the students for self assessment.

I congratulate my student **Dr. NAJMA MOBIN** for her maiden attempt in writing this book which will serve as a useful handbook for students of all health sciences.

With best wishes for future endeavours.

Dr. SHEELA. G. NAYAK

Dean (Academics),

Professor of Anatomy,

KVG Medical College,

Sullia, Dakshina Kannada,

Karnataka,

India.

PREFACE

At the initial stages of medical career every student's difficult subject is understanding anatomy, they feel it's a scary and forgetful phenomena due to new terminologies and find difficult adapting to the new curriculum. As an academician for sixteen years I realized that I have enough knowledge and experience about the subject and should therefore help my students by writing this book and make them to understand that Anatomy is definitely a vast subject but not a difficult one, it can be made fascinating to know and understand the basics of the Human body. I hope this book will help my students to develop passion about the subject. As a mentor I got the feedback from the students saying that they had difficulty in identifying the Histology slides and drawing them in their records, so I thought of solving this problem by offering them nice high resolution pictures in my book. From the exam point of view every chapter in this book starts with the objective and concludes with MCQs and questions asked in the previous exams. At the end of each chapter there is a surgical aspect which is explained in simple language for all the students of pre-clinical and paramedical to understand.

Since this is my maiden book, I humbly request all my students and colleagues to kindly notify if there are any mistakes and omissions in the text.

ACKNOWLEDGEMENTS

I thank the **JSS University**, Mysore, Karnataka, for allowing me to publish this book.

I thank my teacher and senior Professor of Anatomy **Dr. Sheela. G. Nayak**, Dean (Academics), KVG Medical College, Sullia, Dakshina Kannada, Karnataka, for sparing her precious time to write the Foreword for this book.

I wish to express my deepest gratitude to my teacher, guide, mentor and senior Professor of Anatomy **Dr. G. Saraswathi** for her endless support and constant encouragement.

I am very grateful to senior Professor of Anatomy **Dr. N. M. Shama Sundar**, JSS Medical College, Mysore, Karnataka, for his support and immense encouragement.

I thank **Dr. H. BasavanaGowdappa**, Professor and Dean, JSS Medical College, Mysore, Karnataka, for his guidance and support.

I thank **Dr. Pushpalatha. K**, HOD & Professor, Department of Anatomy, JSS Medical College, Mysore, Karnataka, for her support.

I thank **Dr. Priya Ranganath**, Professor and HOD, Department of Anatomy, Bangalore Medical College, Bangalore, and **Dr. Madhu**, Associate Professor, Department of Community Medicine, JSS Medical College, Mysore, Karnataka, for their moral support and encouragement.

I thank my dear colleagues **Dr. Hemamalini, Dr. Vidya.C & Dr. Malar. D** for being supportive.

I thank my beloved husband **Mr. Mohammed Mobin** for giving me his constant support, encouragement and guidance.

I thank the **Notion Press** team for providing me this opportunity to publish this book and giving me guidance in every step of publication.

Chapter 1

INTRODUCTION

The Human Anatomy is the study of structure and functions of various parts of the human body. The term Anatome is a greek word meaning "cutting up." The Gross Anatomy is the study of various structures in the Human body seen with your naked eyes. This can be classified into:

1. **Cadaveric Anatomy:** Study of various systems like cardiovascular system, respiratory system, etc. is known as Systemic anatomy. Study of various regions like upper and lower limbs, thorax, abdomen, etc. is known as regional anatomy. Study of clinical conditions related to a particular region or system is known as Surgical or applied aspects.

2. **Microscopic Anatomy/Histology:** Is study of microscopic structures of various tissues of the body, this is also known as Histology. The tissues are mounted over glass slides and stained with Haematoxylin and Eosin stains and observed under a compound microscope.

3. **Developmental Anatomy/Embryology:** Is the study of developing embryo from the stage of fertilization to a fully developed fetus.

4. **Surface Anatomy:** Is the study of location of various viscera in their normal anatomical positions, by marking over a mummified body.

5. **Radiological Anatomy:** Study of soft tissues, bones and joints using imaging techniques like X-rays, CT-Scan, MRI, etc.

6. **Genetics:** Is study of genes and disorders related to it. Genes are fundamental units of inheritance that are located over the chromosomes.

7. **Applied Anatomy:** Is the study of diseases related to a particular organ or system. The functional and clinical aspects of Anatomy are important for the students to build up their clinical and surgical knowledge.

8. **Sectional Anatomy:** Is study of sections of various parts of the Human body.

9. **Physical Anthrapology:** Study of various parameters of different races and groups of people and also the prehistoric remains.

10. **Comparative Anatomy:** Is the study of comparison between the Human organs with respect to the lower animals, birds, mammals, etc. and study of their structure and functions.

Chapter 2

BASIC ANATOMICAL TERMINOLOGIES

- **Anatomical Position:** The body standing upright with the upper limbs hanging by the sides and the palms facing forwards, with the eyes looking forwards is known as anatomical position.
- **Median Plane:** An imaginary plane that divides the body into two equal halves, right and left.
- **Sagittal Plane:** A plane passing parallel to the median plane.
- **Coronal Plane:** A vertical plane passing at right angles to the median plane.
- **Ventral** (Trunk): (venter = belly) Anything in front of the body;
- **Dorsal** (Trunk): (dorsum = back) Anything behind the body;
- **Anterior:** Nearer the front of the body;
- **Posterior:** Nearer the back of the body;
- **Cephalic/Superior:** Anything nearer to the head;
- **Caudal/Inferior:** Anything nearer to the tail/inferior to the trunk.
- **Medial:** Means nearer to the median plane;
- **Lateral:** Means away from the median plane;
- **Superficial:** Anything nearer to the skin;
- **Deep:** Anything further deeper than the skin;
- **Proximal:** Anything nearer to the root of the structure;
- **Distal:** Anything away from the root of the structure;
- **Palmar:** Related to the palm of the hand;
- **Dorsal**: Related to the dorsum of the hand;
- Combination of terms like superolateral, inferomedial, antero-inferior and postero-superior.

Terminologies Regarding Movements

- **Flexion:** Bending of the limbs anteriorly;
- **Extension:** Bending/straightening of the limbs posteriorly;

- **Adduction:** Movement of the limb towards the median plane;
- **Abduction:** Movement of the limb away from the median plane;
- **Rotation:** Part of the turning around its own longitudinal axis.
- **Supination:** Palm of the hand facing forwards with the elbow joint extended.
- **Pronation:** With the elbow joint extended, the palm facing downwards.
- **Dorsiflexion:** The foot flexed towards the dorsum;
- **Plantarflexion:** The foot extended towards the sole.

Structures to Be Dissected

- **Skin:** The skin consists of epidermis and dermis. The skin is a superficial structure deeper to this lies the muscles and bones.

- **Superficial Fascia:** This is a thin fibrous connective tissue layer separating the skin from the deep fascia. It's dense over the scalp, back of the neck and palm/sole. It is loose over the other parts of the body, this allows free movement of the skin over the underlying structures. It contains arteries, veins, nerves, lymphatics and fat. The fat gives the outer contour of the body and acts as an insulating layer.

- **Deep Fascia:** It is a dense inelastic membrane separating the superficial fascia with the underlying structures. It sends partitions called as **intermuscular septae** inbetween the muscles. It ensheathes the blood vessels and muscles. It forms the outer covering of the bone called as **periosteum.** The retinaculae help to hold the tendons together. It forms **aponeurosis** e.g. epicranial aponeurosis over the scalp, it helps to provide attachments to the muscles. It becomes thickened to form the **ligaments** which are bands of inelastic, white, fibrous tissue connecting the bones especially at the joints.

- **Muscles:** Any muscle has a movable part/end called as **origin** and a fixed part/end called as **insertion.** Each muscle has to be described under the following headings:
  a. **Origin;**
  b. **Insertion;**
  c. **Nerve supply and**
  d. **Action.**

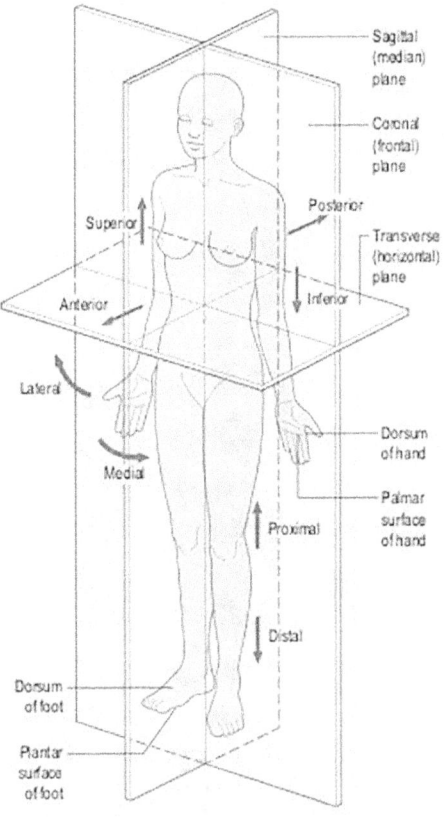

Anatomical Planes: 1

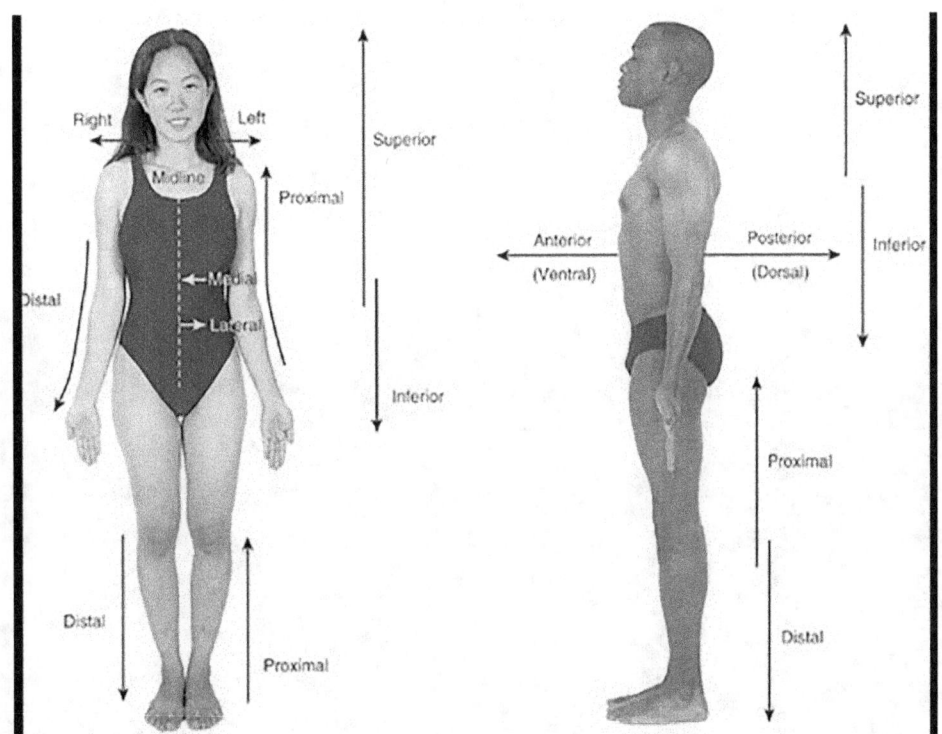

Anatomical Terminologies: 2

<h1 style="text-align:center">Chapter 3</h1>

<h1 style="text-align:center">SUPERFICIAL AND DEEP FASCIA</h1>

Objectives of This Topic

1. To understand the structure, contents and functions of superficial and deep fascia.
2. To identify the various modifications of the deep fascia while performing dissection.
3. To obtain knowledge about their surgical importance.

Superficial Fascia

Definition: The collection of connective tissue below the skin, in between the muscles and bones is known as fascia, which can be superficial or deep. The superficial layer is made up of loose areolar connective tissue while the deep layer is quite dense and inelastic membrane. Quality of adipose tissue is superficial fascia varies from region to region.

Distribution of Adipose Tissue

1. Due to uniform distribution of fat in females, they have a rounded contour as compared to males.
2. Minimum adipose tissue is seen over dorsum of hands and feet.
3. Abundant fat is located over the gluteal region (buttocks), lower abdominal area and mammary gland in females.
4. The fibrous mesh of superficial fascia is very dense over the scalp, palm and sole.
5. There is no fat over the eyelids, nipples, areola of mammary gland, ear, penis and scrotum.

Contents of Superficial Fascia

1. It contains nerves, blood vessels and lymphatics.
2. It may contain lower ends of sweat glands in the skin.
3. It may also contain subcutaneous muscles like the dartos muscle of the scrotum and palmaris brevis in the palm.

Functions of Superficial Fascia

1. It conserves body heat, thus acts as an insulating agent deep to the skin. The veins in the fascia contract during cold weather causing less blood flow, whereas the veins dilate in hot weather so that heat is lost from the blood as seen while sweating.

2. It acts as a binding agent and binds the nerves and blood vessels together and provides easy passage.

3. It acts as a cushion for fragile structures underneath.

4. It provides energy storehouse as seen in the sites like buccal pad of fat and gluteal fat.

5. It forms a firm platform holding the skin with the deep fascia as seen over the palm and sole.

Deep Fascia

Definition: It is dense type of inelastic connective tissue made up of regularly arranged collagen fibres and lies just beneath the superficial fascia. It converts the muscles and blood vessels of almost the whole body except for few regions like face. It is very sensitive due to rich nerve supply.

Modifications of Deep Fascia

a. **Retinaculum and Fibrous Flexors Sheaths:** The deep fascia becomes thickened to hold the tendons together as the joints together, these are transverse bands of dense connective tissue.

    Example: Seen around the wrist, ankle, and joints. They form osteo-fibrous tunnels through which various tendons and nerves pass. The retinacula act as pulleys wherein, the tendons may move easily and can change their directions. The fibrous flexors sheaths are thickened fascia seen over the fingers and toes of the flexor surface, these sheaths help to retain the flexor tendons in position during flexion of interphalangeal joints thus preventing bowing out of position.

b. **Aponeurosis:** These are localized sheet of dense, thick fibrous tissue through which muscles are attached.

    Example: Palmar and plantar aponeuroses of hand and foot. These sheets of fibrous tissue protect the deep or underlying structures like nerves, blood vessels and tendons of various muscles. The palmar aponeurosis receives insertion of palmaris longus muscle. The bicipital aponeurosis of biceps brachii muscles forms the roof of cubital fossa which helps as a platform for giving intravenous injections. The iliotibial tract seen over the lateral aspect of the thighs provides attachments to two muscles are tensor fascia latae and gluteus maximus muscles.

c. **Ligaments:** These are long thick modified deep fascia connecting the bones at the joints, these band - like structures are made up of bundles of collagen fibers, therefore, inelastic they just hold the bones in position during joint movements.

d. **Inter-Muscular Septa:** These are sheets of fibrous tissue seen in between the muscles as seen in upper and lower limbs dividing the limbs into components like flexor and extensor compartments. These are attached to the bones, thus limit the spread of infection or tumour. It provides additional attachment to the muscles.

e. **Musculo-Nervous Pumps:** The deep fascia seen in the limbs provide outwards expansion like a sleeve during muscular contractions, they compress the intra-muscular veins which helps the venous blood to return to the heart, thus forming musculo-venous pumps as seen in the soleus muscles in the calf or back to the leg. The soleus is also called as "peripheral heart." The back flow of the blood is prevented by the venous valves.

f. Deep cervical fascia in the neck forms partitions in the neck region thus limiting the spread of infection.

Functions of the Deep Fascia

1. It forms musculo-venous pump thus helping in venous return.
2. It provides muscular attachments.
3. Through its modifications it protects the underlying structures like aponeurosis.
4. It stabilizes the joints through ligaments.
5. The retinacular and flexor sheaths provide change in direction to tendons and smooth gliding movements over the joints.
6. The muscular partitions prevent the spread of infection from over compartment to another.

g. **Sheaths:** These are shot sleeve like fibrous partitions seen in the thigh like femoral sheath and in the neck like carotid sheath. These sheaths act as protective covering for important blood vessels and nerves. They provide easy passage for the vessels and nerves.

Multiple Choice Questions

1. The following are modifications of deep fascia except:
   a. Aponeurosis.
   b. Inter-muscular septa.
   c. Retinacular.
   d. Fascia of face.
   (Answer: d)

2. All of the following are functions of deep fascia except:
   a. It forms musculo-venous pump.
   b. It provides muscular attachments.
   c. It provides friction and tenses the tendons.
   d. It stabilizes joints through ligaments.
   (Answer: c)

Model Questions

Write Short Notes On

1. Superficial fascia-distributions and functions.
2. Deep fascia modifications and functions.

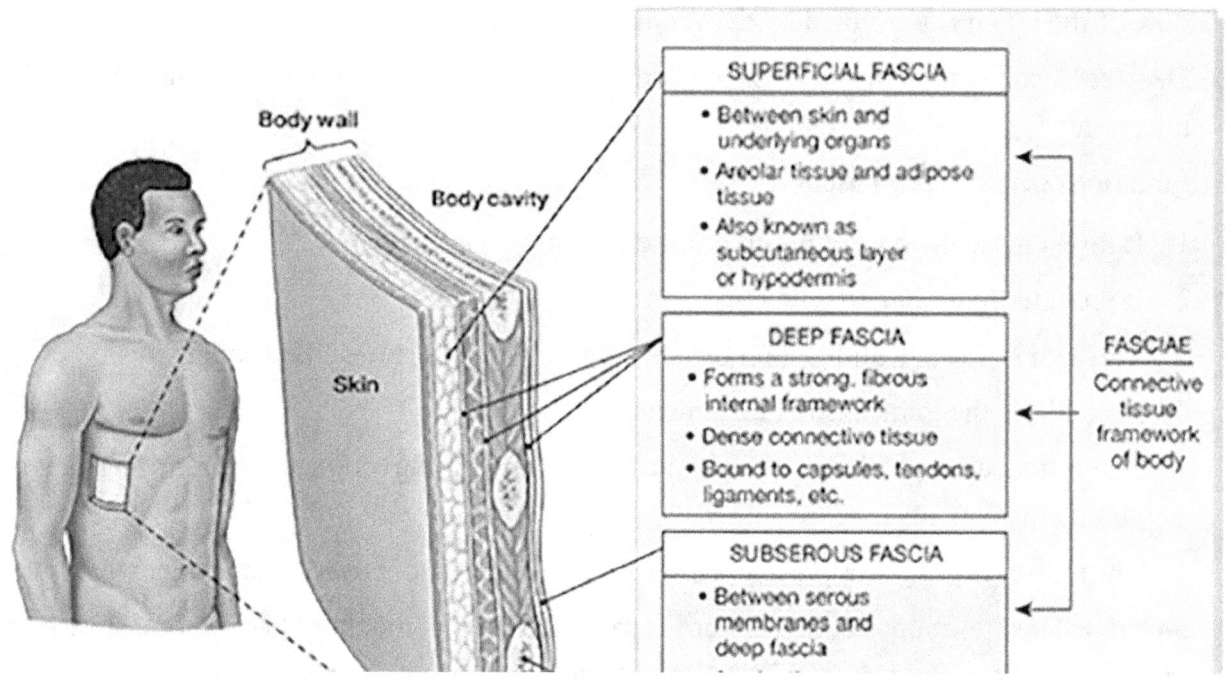

Fascia: 1

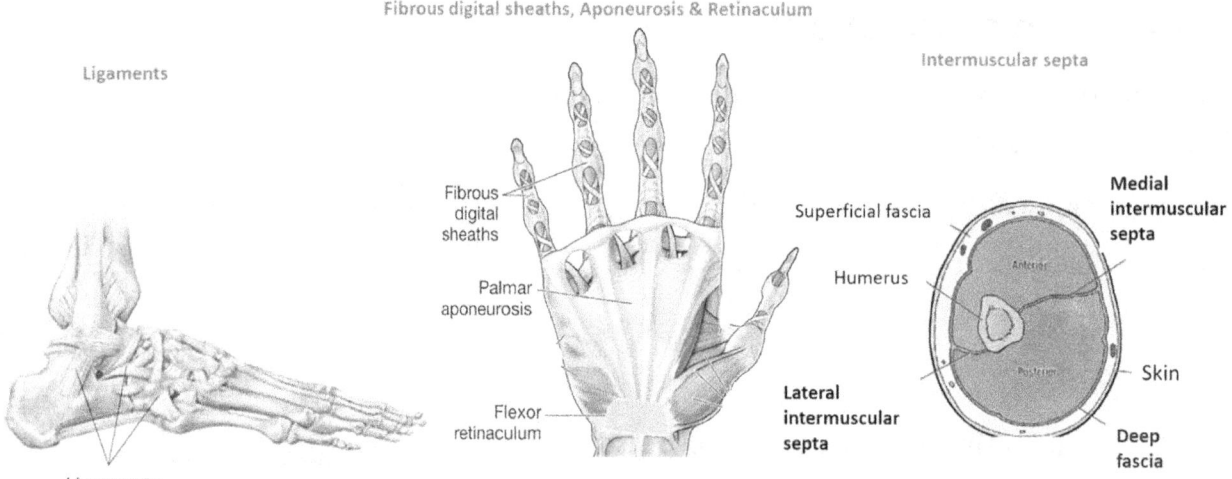

Fascia: 2

Chapter 4

CELLS AND CELL DIVISION

Objectives

1. The basic constituent of various types of cells is important to know their functional aspects and their normal appearance.

2. The steps involved in cell division are necessary to know in order to understand various genetic disorders.

   Cells are basic structural and functional units of the body.

   Somatic cells are essential for growth, development and regeneration.

   Whereas, germ cells are essential for production of gametes.

   Somatic cells have 23 pairs of chromosomes (diploid)-female-xx and male-xy. Gametes have 23 chromosomes (haploid).

Constituents of a Cell

Cell membrane/Plasma membrane – Covering of a cell;

Nucleus – Contains genetic material of the cell;

Cytoplasm – Watery fluid containing cell organelles like mitochondria, endoplasmic reticulum, ribosomes, Golgi apparatus, etc.

Plasma membrane – Consists of two layers of phospholipids and protein molecules, each phospholipid molecule has a hydrophilic head and a hydrophobic tail.

Functions of Plasma Membrane

- Provides cell immunity;
- Act as receptors for hormones and chemical messengers, some act as enzymes;
- Helps to transport chemical substances across the membrane.

NUCLEUS: Contains Nucleolus and nucleoplasm, the genetic material contains DNA and HISTONES (proteins)which make up the chromatin threads and form a network of chromosomes, the functional unit of this is gene. The nucleolus contains RNA and proteins.

Cell Organelles

MITOCHONDRIA: Are power houses of the cell, involved in aerobic respiration wherein, the chemical energy is released in form of ATP.

Metabolically active cells like muscle cells and liver cells contain numerous mitochondria since the energy released is very high. Inner membrane is folded and contains enzymes, RNA and DNA.

Endoplasmic Reticulum

* **Rough ER** – Contains the ribosomes and are the sites of protein synthesis.
* **Smooth ER** – Devoid of ribosomes and are the sites of lipid synthesis and secrete steroids.
* The **ribosomes** help in protein synthesis and contain RNA, singly called as monosome and in group called as polysomes.

GOLGI APPARATUS: Made up of closely binded flat membranous sacs, it's the site of processing and packaging of proteins synthesized by the ER. The proteins are stored in the vesicles (secretory granules).

Lysosomes

* Dense bodies containing acid hydrolase which destroys the unwanted material from the cell by intra cytoplasmic digestion.
* They bring about phagocytosis of bacteria/viruses, thereby called as "suicidal bags of the cell."
* Centrioles: Rod like structures lying close to the nucleus, made up of microtubules, play an important role in cell division and formation of cellular structures like cilia and flagella.
* Cytoplasmic inclusion bodies: membrane bound vesicles containing bacteria, melanin, lipids, etc.

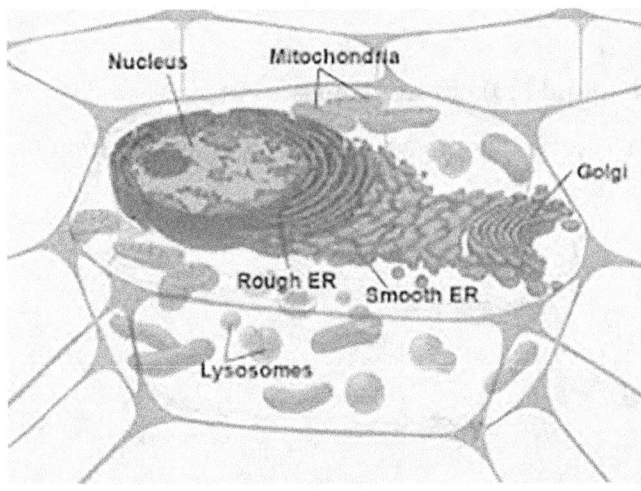

Cell Organelle: 1

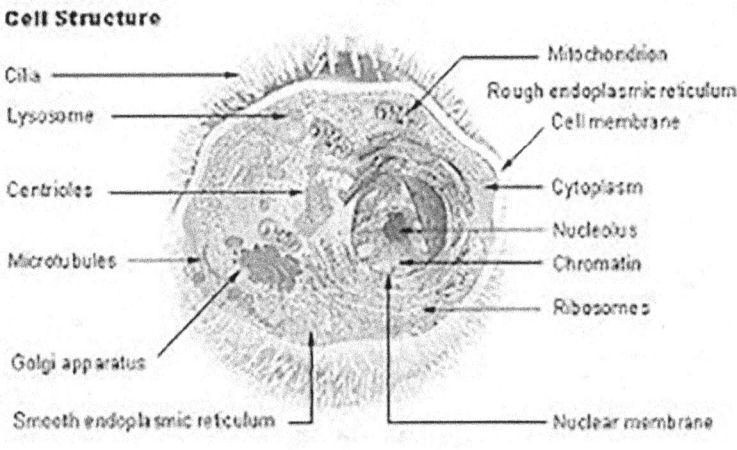

Cell Organelle: 2

Cell Division

Mitosis

Omatic cells divide by mitosis and daughter cells have diploid number of chromosomes (2n). DNA content duplicates and another chromatid is formed.

- **Prophase** – Chromatin gets coiled, centrioles separate, microtubules are formed and help in spindle formation, nucleolus disappears and nuclear membrane breaks.

- **Metaphase** – Chromosomes arrange at equator, attached to microtubules of spindle by the centromere.

- **Anaphase** – Centromeres of all the chromatids divide longitudinally and the two chromatids become independent chromosomes. Each cell has 46 pairs of chromosomes. One chromosome from each pair migrates to either pole of the cell along the spindle.

- **Telophase** – The daughter cell covered by cell membrane, chromosomes elongate, nucleoli reappear, and centrioles duplicate.

Meiosis

◆ Daughter cells have haploid (23) chromosomes.

◆ First meiotic division – Leptotene; zygotene; pachytene; diplotene.

◆ Second meiotic division-Same as mitosis.

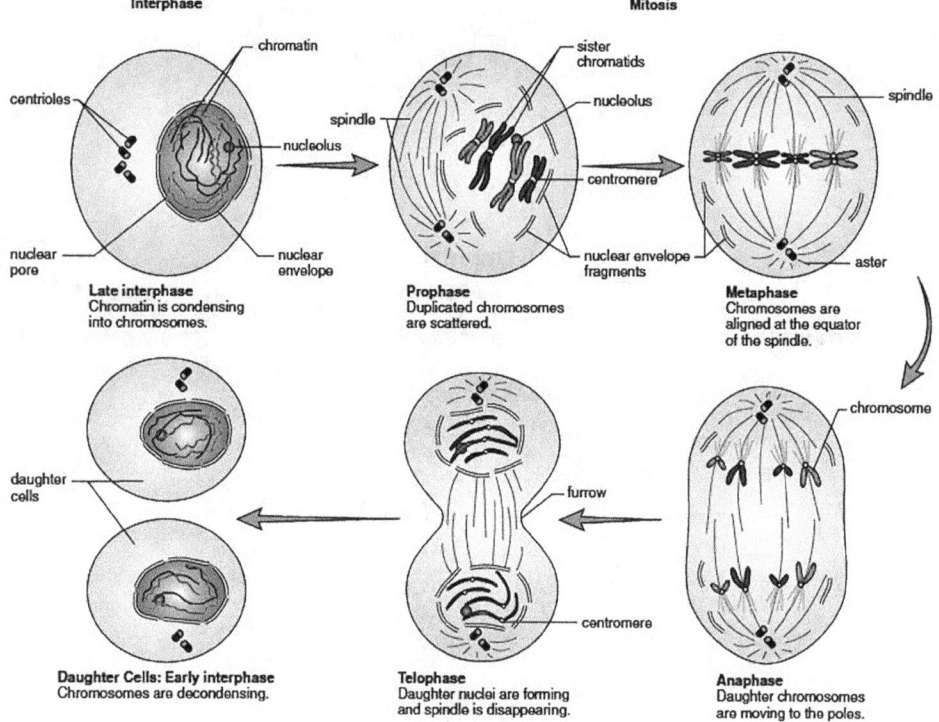

Cell Division: 1

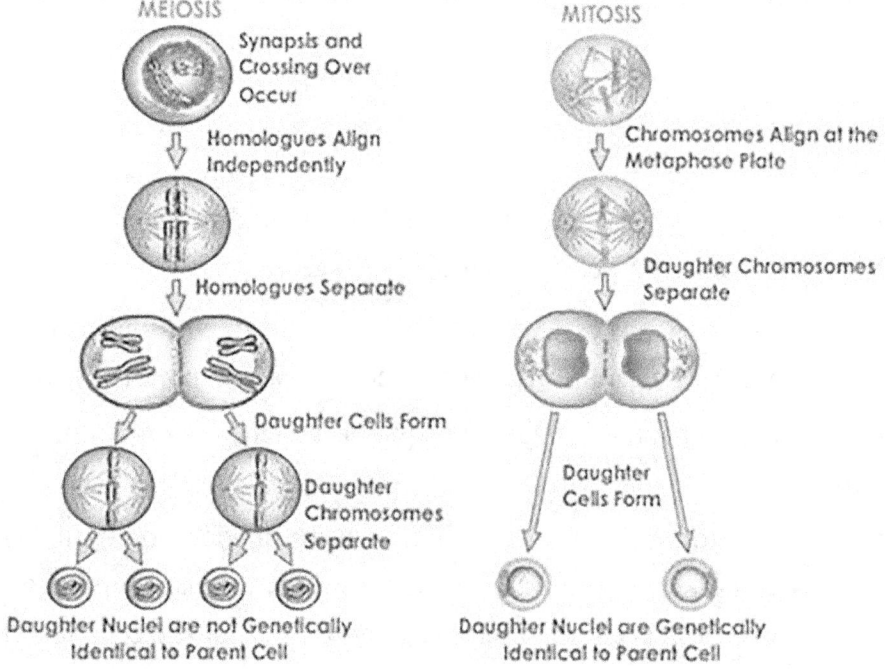

Cell Division: 2

Multiple Choice Questions

1. "Suicidal bags of the cell" is:

   a. Mitochondria;

   b. Lysosomes;

   c. Golgi apparatus;

   d. Endoplasmic reticulum.

   (Answer: b)

2. Chromosomes arrange at equator, attached to microtubules of spindle by the centromere, in which phase:

   a. Telophase;

   b. Metaphase;

   c. Anaphase;

   d. Prophase.

   (Answer: b)

Model Questions

Short Notes (5 Marks)

1. Write the functions of Mitochondria.
2. Write the structure and functions of Endoplasmic reticulum.
3. Write the functions of lysosomes.

Chapter 5

EPITHELIAL TISSUE

Objective

The normal microscopic tissue lining must be known in order to know the abnormal tissue components and diseases related to the tissues.

Definition: Tissue is defined as a collection of cells along with the intercellular substance and performing the same function. The epithelial tissue covers the body surface and lines the hollow tubular structures.

Important Characteristic Features of Epithelial Tissues

- The cells are closely packed together;
- The cells rest over a basement membrane;
- There are NO capillaries, nutrition is derived from the nearby capillaries;
- Surface cells get destroyed by wear and tear, the cells get replaced by mitosis (turn over).

Functions of Epithelial Tissues

- **Protection:** Skin protects the body from external environment;
- **Secretion:** Goblet cells present in the gastrointestinal tract and respiratory tract secrete mucus, which protects and decreases friction;
- **Absorption:** Epithelium lining the gastrointestinal tract helps in absorption and digestion;
- **Lubrication:** Serous cavities like the pleural, pericardial and peritoneal cavities are lined with a thin film of capillary fluid which lubricate and prevent the separation of layers.

Classification of Epithelium

I.   **SIMPLE EPITHELIUM:** Lined with a single layer of cells which lie over a basement membrane. It is present where the absorption is more, & wear and tear is less. It consists of:

a.   *Simple squamous epithelium (for figure refer page no. 66)*: The cells are flat resting over a thin basement membrane. The cells have a flat nucleus and appear like a pavement.

Functions: These help in dialyzing or filtering substances as in the tubules of nephrons; exchange of gases as in the alveoli of lungs; secretion in the serous cavities for lubrication; expansion of blood vessels.

Examples: Lining of lung alveoli; lining of serous cavities (mesothelium); lining of blood vessels (endothelium).

b.   *Simple cuboidal epithelium (for figure refer page no. 66):* It is a single layer of cubical cells lying over a basement membrane. The cells have round nucleus.

Functions: These help mainly in secretion.

Examples: Follicles of thyroid; follicles of prostate, etc.

c.   *Simple columnar epithelium (for figure refer page no. 67):* The cells are tall column like with oval nucleus, lying over a basement membrane. Some show vertical striations called as brush border epithelium, these are small microvilli and are seen in PCT of nephrons and small & large intestines. The cells that have filamentous thread like structures are called as ciliated epithelium, which may be motile/non motile, the non motile cilia are called as stereocilia.

Functions: Mainly secretion and absorption. The brush border helps in active absorption and increase the surface area. The cilia help in the transport of substances and protection. The stereocilia help to increase the surface area of mucous membrane.

Examples: Columnar cells are seen in the gastrointestinal tract; ciliated epithelium is seen the respiratory tract; uterine tubes and auditory tube. Stereocilia are seen in ventricles of the brain and spinal cord; epididymis; etc.

d.   *Pseudo stratified epithelium (for figure refer page no. 67)*: Pseudo means false, therefore, there's false appearance of stratification but actually it's a single layer of cells. Some of the cells are small and some are tall therefore, the nuclei lie at different levels giving a false appearance of stratification.

Functions: Secretion and absorption of substances.

Examples of pseudo stratified ciliated epithelium are mucous membrane of nasal cavity, trachea and bronchi.

Other types of cells: Goblet cells: Are modified columnar cells and contain mucus secreted by the rough endoplasmic reticulum, stored and excreted by Golgi apparatus, e.g. Gastrointestinal tract and respiratory tract.

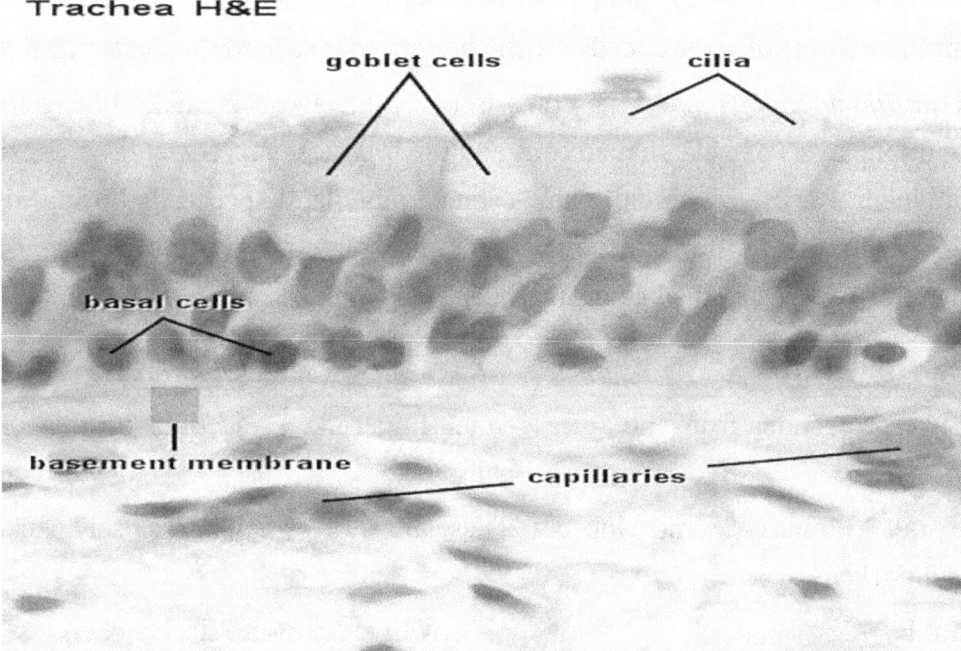

Pseudostratified Epithelium: 5

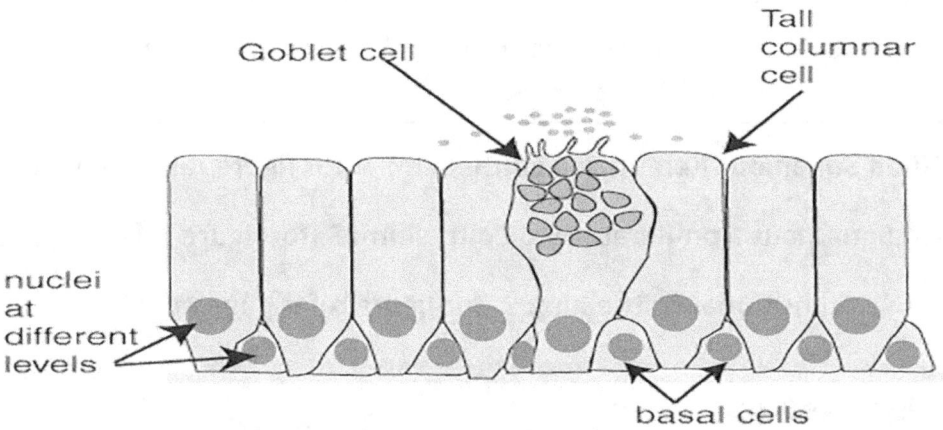

Pseudostratified Epithelium: 6

II. **COMPOUND EPITHELIUM:** This is of two types: Stratified and Transitional epithelia.

1. The stratified epithelium consists of stratified columnar, stratified squamous and stratified cuboidal epithelia.

    a. *Stratified columnar epithelium*: Consists of multiple layers of cells.

    Examples: Male urethra.

    b. *Stratified squamous epithelium*: This consists of basal layer of columnar cells, over which there are multiple layers of polyhedral cells, the most superficial layers consists of squamous cells. The top most layers may be keratinized (cornified) or non keratinized.

    Examples: Keratinized is seen in the epidermis of thick skin; non keratinized is seen in oral cavity, tongue, oesophagus, vagina, lower part of anal canal and cornea.

c. *Stratified cuboidal epithelium*: This consists of basal layer of small cells, over which lie multiple layers of cubical cells. Such epithelium is seen in the ducts of salivary glands.

d. *Transitional epithelium:* This consists of basal layer of small cells, over which lie multiple layers of pear shaped cells and the top most superficial layer consists of large polyhedral cells, which can change into umbrella shaped cells during distension of the organ. Such a transition of epithelium is seen in the urinary bladder and ureters therefore, it's also called as urothelium.

CILIA	MICROVILLI
Small hair-like projections from the apices of the cells.	Small finger-like projections on the apices of the cells.
These are tall, elongated and loosely arranged and packed.	These are short, small and closely packed.
Cilia are motile.	Microvilli are non-motile.
Rich in microtubules (9 × 2).	Rich in microfilaments.
Seen under the ordinary microscope.	Seen only under electron microscope.
Help to entrap the foreign particles like dust.	Help in absorption of nutrients.

Stratified Squamous Keratinized Epithelium: 7 (for figure refer page no. 68)

Stratified Squamous Non-Keratinized Epithelium: 8 (for figure refer page no. 68)

Transitional Epithelium: 9 (for figure refer page no. 69)

Types of Epithelium

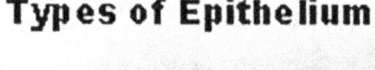
Simple squamous

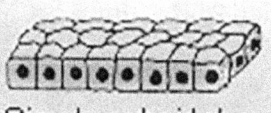
Simple cuboidal

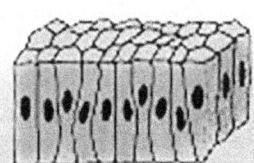
Simple columnar

Transitional

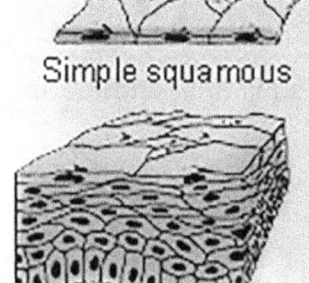
Stratified squamous

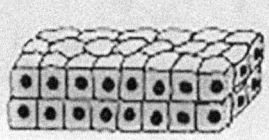
Stratified cuboidal

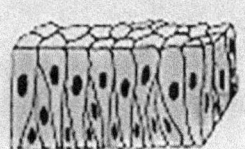
Pseudostratified columnar

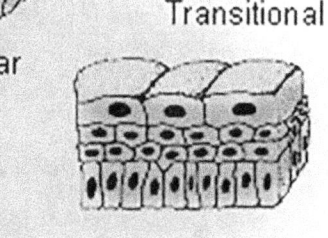

Epithelium: 10

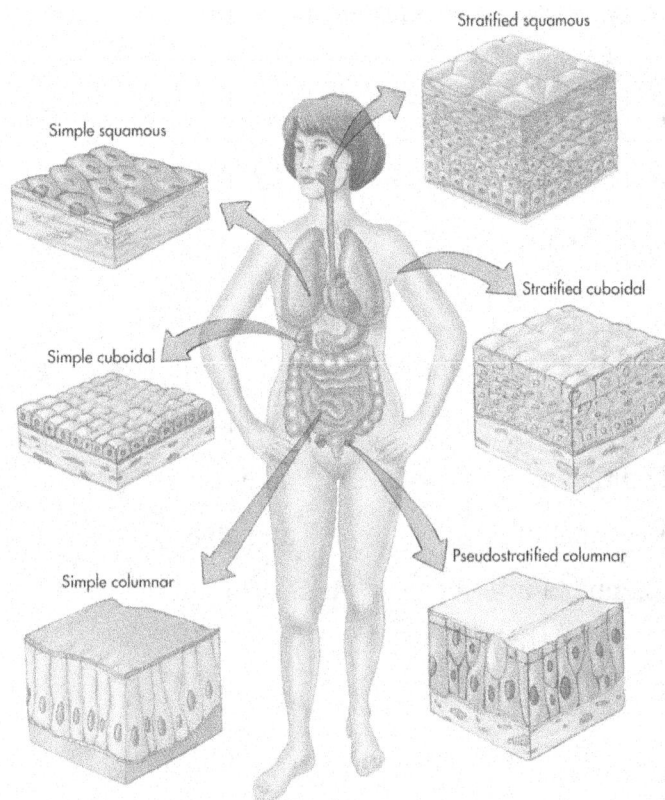

Epithelium: 11

Multiple Choice Questions

1. Stratified squamous non- kertinized epithelium is seen in all of the following except:

    a. Thick skin;

    b. Vagina;

    c. Oesophagus;

    d. Oral cavity.

    (Answer: a)

2. All of the following statements is true except:

    a. Cilia are motile;

    b. Cilia are small finger-like projections on the apices of the cells.

    c. Cilia help to entrap foreign particles.

    d. Cilia are rich in micro tubules.

    (Answer: b)

3. The following features of Endothelium is true except:

    a. It lines the peritoneal cavity;

    b. It lines the blood vessels;

    c. It is simple squamous type of epithelium;

    d. It permits exchange of nutrients.

    (Answer: a)

4. Match the following Epithelium with their examples:

    i.   Pseudostratified epithelium   a. Thyroid follicles;

    ii. Simple Cuboidal epithelium   b. Trachea;

    iii. Simple Columnar epithelium   c. Lung alveoli;

    iv. Simple Squamous epiyhelium   d. Gastro-intestinal tract.

    (Answer: i (b); ii (a); iii (d); iv (c))

Model Questions

Main Question (10 Marks)

1. Classify epithelium giving examples for each.

Short Notes (5 Marks)

1. Describe the transitional epithelium giving examples.

Short Answers (2 Marks)

1. Describe Simple squamous epithelium with examples.

Chapter 6

CONNECTIVE TISSUE

Objectives

1. The different types of cells and fibres their structure and functions in connective tissues are important in order to differentiate them from abnormal cells and fibres in different pathological conditions.

2. Loose and dense type of connective tissues are basic tissues holding the body frame work together, therefore requires detailed knowledge about their structure and functions.

The Connective Tissue Is of Two Types

1. **Loose Connective Tissue:** Consists of loose areolar connective tissue and adipose tissue.

2. **Dense Connective Tissue:** Consists of bone and cartilage.

   The connective tissue components include the various types of cells, fibres and ground matrix.

FIBRES: These are of three types namely: Collagen, elastic and reticular fibres.

1. **Collagen Fibres:** Here the fibres run in wavy bundles, and are formed by the fibroblasts, the bundles show branching pattern.

   Types of Collagen Fibres

   - **Type 1** – Bone, tendon, ligaments, dermis and dentine;
   - **Type 2** – Hyaline cartilage;
   - **Type 3** – Smooth muscles of GIT, CVS and Uterus;
   - **Type 4** – Basement membrane.

2. **Elastic Fibres:** These are single, isolated, having twisted ends, and form a network, they retract and recoil. They are formed by the fibroblasts.

3. **Reticular Fibres:** These are finely branched fibres forming a network. They are seen in liver and bone marrow. They are also formed by the reticular cells/fibroblasts.

Cells of Connective Tissue

◆ **Fibroblasts:** These are stem cells; spindle shaped, they produce and maintain fibres and the ground substance.

◆ **Fat Cells:** These cells help in the synthesis of fat and its storage. Their nucleus is flat with clear cytoplasm (signet ring appearance), it's present in the adipose tissue of breast, cheek and buttocks.

◆ **Macrophages:** These are irregular cells with oval nucleus; they phagocytose bacteria by engulfing the particles, the lysosomes then digest these materials.

◆ **Plasma Cells:** The plasma cells develop immunity in the body, and are seen in the lymphatic tissues and loose areolar tissue. They cells are rounded with cart-wheel appearance of the nucleus. The antibodies are formed by these cells. They develop from the B-Lymphocytes.

◆ **Mast Cells:** The mast cells are round cells having oval nucleus, cytoplasm has granules with histamine/heparin. Histamine produces allergy and heparin is an anticoagulant.

◆ **Lymphocytes:** Two types-B and T-Lymphocytes. B-lymphocytes produce antibodies (humoral immunity), T-lymphocytes help in cell-mediated immunity.

Ground Substance: The ground substance/matrix is made up of acid glycosaminoglycans (AGAG), proteoglycans and water, e.g. Heparan in liver, chondroitin sulphate in cartilage, dermatan in skin, keratan in cornea, etc.

Functions of Matrix/Ground Substance

◆ Maintains framework/morphology of tissues;

◆ Protects and binds the CT cells;

◆ Acts as a mechanical barrier;

◆ Helps in diffusion of metabolites;

◆ Helps in storage of water.

Loose Areolar Tissue: 1 (for figure refer page no. 69)

This is made up of fibres, different types of cells and ground substance. It's present in sub-cutaneous tissue, sub-mucous coat of GIT, Sub-serous coat of tissues, around the blood vessels and muscles, etc.

Loose Areolar Tissue: 2 (for figure refer page no. 70)

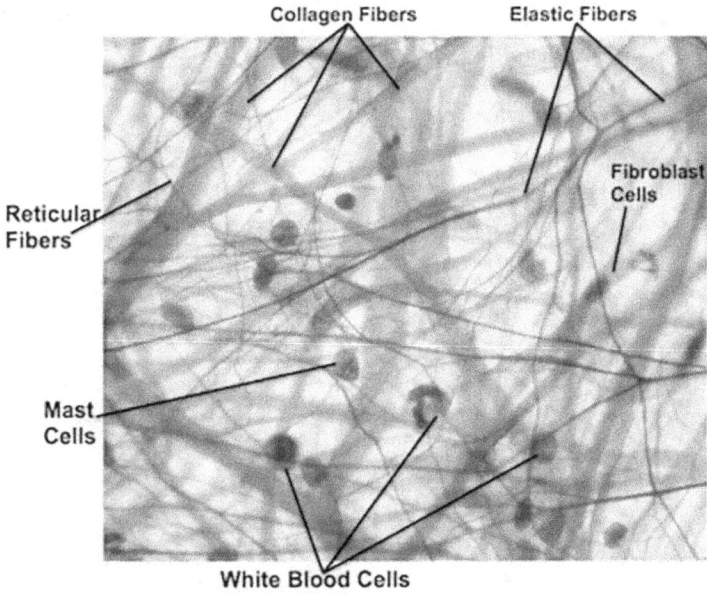

Loose Areolar Tissue: 3

ADIPOSE TISSUE: It's made up of fat cells or adipocytes, contains enzymes that help in fatty acid synthesis from glucose, e.g. Buccal pad of fat in the cheek, gluteal fat/buttocks, around the kidneys, anterior abdominal wall, etc. It has poor blood supply. It may have unilocular or mutilocular adipocytes.

FUNCTIONS OF ADIPOSE TISSUE: Storehouse of fat, acts as a cushion, conserves body heat, provides a packing material around the viscera, and maintains the contour of the body.

Adipose Tissue: 4 (for figure refer page no. 70)

Adipose Tissue: 5 (for figure refer page no. 71)

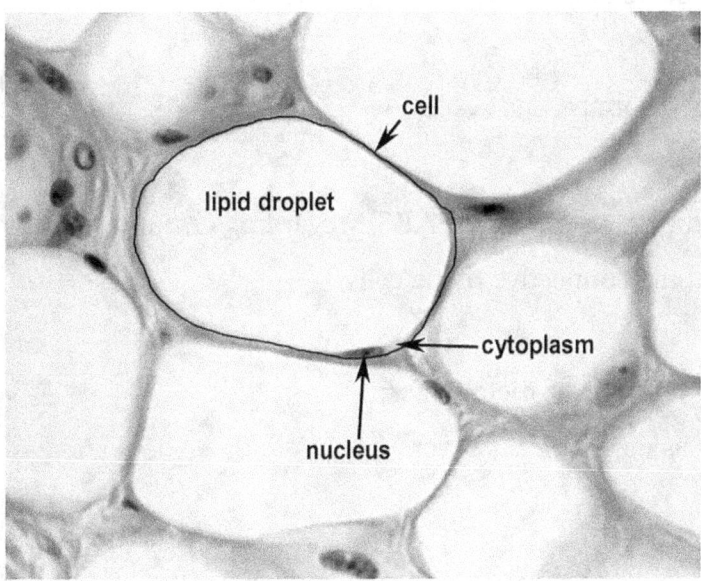

Adipose Tissue: 6

TENDON: It's made up of bundles of collagen fibres, which run parallel to each other, the matrix is very less, and the tendon cells are called as tenocytes.

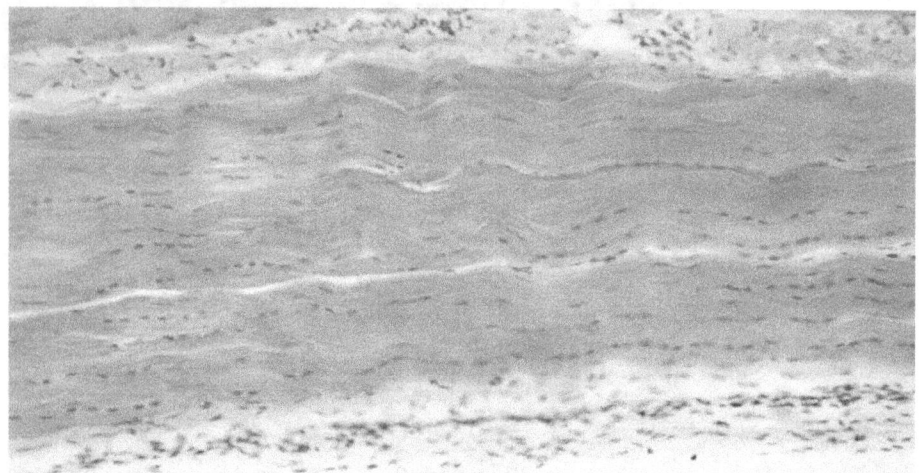

Tendon: 7

Applied Anatomy

1. Disorders related to collagen fibres are: Scleroderma; Rheumatoid arthritis, etc.

2. Marfan's syndrome is an inherited disorder leading to abnormal multiplication of Elastic fibres due to defective fibrillin gene, features like tall stature, long fingers/toes, etc. are seen.

Multiple Choice Questions

1. Regarding Adipose tissue which of the following statements are TRUE except:

   a. It contains unilocular or multilocular adipocytes;

   b. It does not conserve body heat;

   c. It is seen in buttocks;

   d. It has poor blood supply.

   (Answer: b)

2. Which of the following statement is FALSE regarding Ground substance:

   a. It helps to bind the connective tissue cells;

   b. It stores water;

   c. It helps in the diffusion of metabolites;

   d. It does not act as mechanical barrier.

   (Answer: d)

3. Type II Collagen fibres are seen in:

   a. White fbro cartilage;

   b. Elastic cartilage;

   c. Hyaline cartlage;

   d. All of the above.

   (Answer: c)

Model Questions

Short Notes (5 Marks)

1. Histology of loose areolar tissue with a neat labelled diagram.

2. Histology of adipose tissue with a neat labelled diagram.

Short Answers (2 Marks)

1. Name the cells and fibres in the loose areolar tissue.

2. Name the components of connective tissue.

Chapter 7

CARTILAGE

Objectives of This Topic

1. To know the normal microscopic picture of different types of cartilages.
2. To differentiate normal from abnormal appearances as seen in conditions like osteoarthritis, rheumatoid arthritis, slip disc etc.
3. To know the sites and functions of various types of cartilages.

Dense/Regular Connective Tissue

1. Fibrous connective tissue.
   a. Tendons.
   b. Ligaments.
2. Rigid connective tissue.
   a. Cartilage-three types.
      i. Hyaline cartilage.
      ii. Elastic cartilage.
      iii. White-fibro cartilage.

Definition of Cartilage

"Cartilage is a specialized modified form of dense connective tissue which is designed to provide support bear weight and to withstand tension, torsion and bending."

Functions of Cartilage

1. To support the body that requires flexibility and resistance.
2. To provide a framework.
3. To protect underlying fragile structures.

4. To provide muscular attachments.

5. To structural model for growing bones.

General Features of Cartilage

1. Cartilage is non nervous structure, therefore insensitive.

2. When cartilage is connected with bone through calcification, then it can be temporary or permanent cartilage.

3. The fetal skeleton is made up of temporary hyaline cartilage which later becomes calcified to form bones.

4. Cartilage has poor regenerating capacity any defects is usually filled up by fibrous tissue.

5. It does not have blood vessels or lymphatics, it receives its nutrition by peripheral capillaries or vessels in the perichondrium through diffusion.

6. Only the hyaline cartilage undergoes calcification, seen especially in the old age.

Perichondrium

1. The cartilage is covered externally by perichondrium (except the articular cartilages and white-fibro cartilage).

2. It is made up of outer fibrous layer and inner cellular layer/chondrogenic layer.

Major Components of Cartilage

1. Cells called as chondrocytes which are mature cells and chondroblasts which are immature cells.

2. Fibers-collagen or elastic.

3. Ground substance or matrix made up of mucopolysaccharides like chondroitinsulphate, keratin sulphate and hyaluronic acid. Glycosaminoglycan (GAG), proteins and proteoglycans.

Cell of Cartilages/Chondrocytes

1. They are derived from undifferentiated mesenchymal cells.

2. Young and immature cells with branched cytoplastic process are known as chondroblasts, which later multiply into chondrocytes.

3. Chondrocytes are larger in size surrounded by space known as lacunae.

4. They produce the fibers and matrix of the cartilage.

5. Old mature cells do not multiply.

Development and Growth of Cartilage

The cartilage grows by two methods:

1. Appositional growth.
2. Interstitial growth.

Appositional Growth

Here the new cartilage cells grow over the surface of existing cartilage the osteogenic layer of the perichondrium helps in the growth of cartilage, here the fibroblasts divide and gets differentiated into chondroblasts, these cells are surrounded by matrix and then are converted into mature cells called as chondrocytes. Finally, the matrix gets deposited below the perichondrium over the outer surface of cartilage thus, making it to grow in width.

Interstitial Growth

The cartilage grows by the cells that constantly multiply within the substance of the cartilage. The cells synthesize the new matrix thus expanding the cartilage within itself therefore, known as "interstitial."

Types of Cartilages

Hyaline Cartilage: 1 (for figure refer page no. 71)

a. This has perichondrium and characterized by highly basophilic homogeneous matrix.
b. The homogenicity is due to the same refractive index of the collagen fibres and the ground substance.
c. The cells are arranged in groups and surrounded by the space called as lacuna and the cells are encapsulated.
d. The group of cells are called as "cell **nests**," which are characteristic of hyaline cartilage.
e. The matrix around the cell **nests** is brighter and more basophilic and is known as "territorial matrix."
f. The lightly coloured matrix is between the cell **nests** is known as "inter-territorial matrix."

Examples of hyaline cartilages:

  i. Costal cartilages.
  ii. Articular cartilages.
  iii. Tracheal rings.

The articular cartilages are devoid of perichondrium.

Elastic Cartilage: 2 (for figure refer page no. 72)

a. Also known as yellow fibro-cartilage.

b. Perichondrium is present.

c. The matrix shows numerous elastic fibres which branch and anastomose.

d. Chondrocytes are isolated dispersed surrounded by lacunae.

e. They are larger in size.

  Examples:

     i. Ear/pinna/auricle.

    ii. Epiglottis.

   iii. Eustachian tube/external auditory canal.

White-Fibrocartilage: 3 (for figure refer page no. 72)

a. There is no perichondrium.

b. It has thick bundles of collagen fibers.

c. The chondrocytes are single and arranged in a row in between the bundles of collagen fibers.

  Examples:

      i. Pubic symphysis.

     ii. Intervartebral discs.

    iii. Manubriosternal joint.

    iv. Glenoidal labrum.

     v. Acetabular labrum.

Hyaline Cartilage: 4 (for figure refer page no. 73)

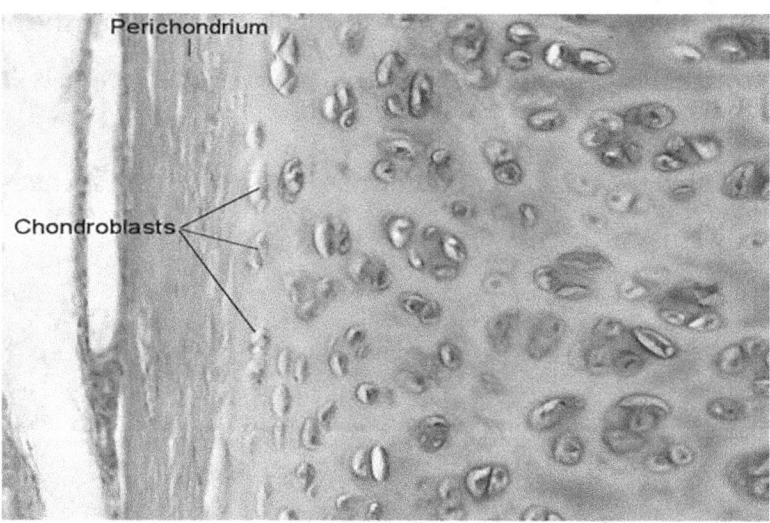

Hyaline Cartilage: 5

Elastic Cartilage: 6 (for figure refer page no. 73)

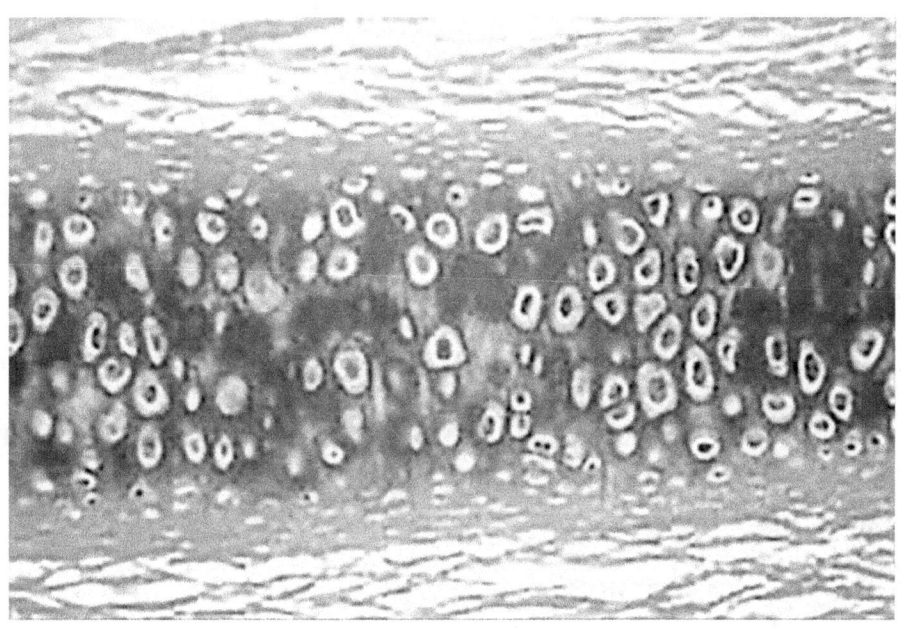

Elastic Cartilage: 7

White Fibro – Cartilage: 8 (for figure refer page no. 74)

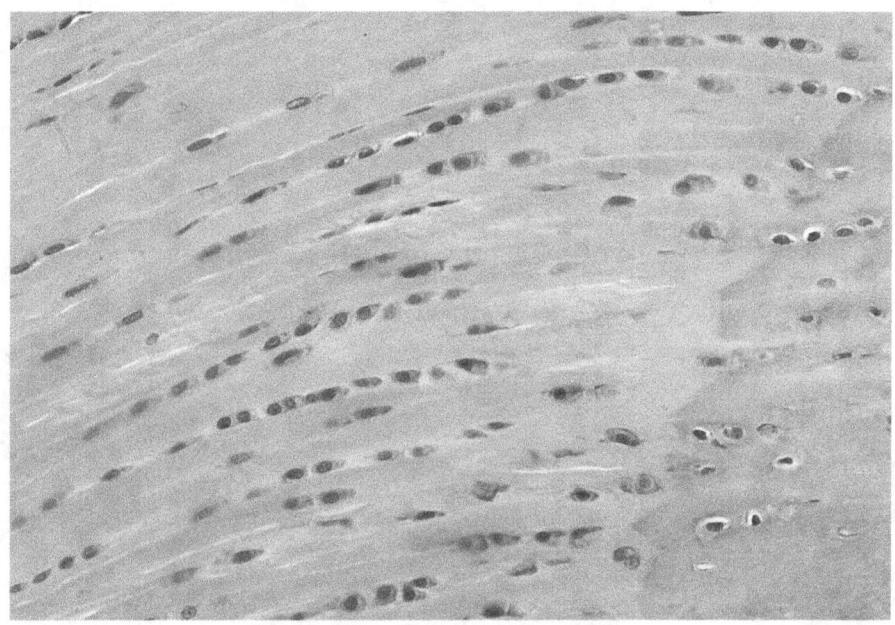

White Fibro – Cartilage: 9

Applied Anatomy

1. Osteoarthritis.

2. Slip disc.

3. Hyaline cartilage has tendency to ossify with age.

4. Rheumatoid arthritis.

Multiple Choice Questions

1. Hyaline cartilage is characteristic of:
   a. Abundant elastic fibers.
   b. Isolated chondrocytes.
   c. Cell nests.
   d. Devoid of perichondrium.
   (Answer: d)

2. Elastic cartilage is present in all of the following except:
   a. Auricle.
   b. Epiglottis.
   c. Esophagus.
   d. Eustachian tube.
   (Answer: c)

3. Perichondrium is not seen in:
   a. Hyaline cartilage.
   b. Elastic cartilage.
   c. White fibro-cartilage.
   d. Yellow cartilage.
   (Answer: c)

4. The "ground-glass" appearance of the matrix in hyaline cartilage is due to:
   a. Chondroitin sulphate.
   b. Keratan sulphate.
   c. Reticular fibres.
   d. Elastic fibres.
   (Answer: a)

Model Questions

Write Short Notes On (5 Marks Each)

1. Describe the Hyaline cartilage with the help of a neat labeled diagram.
2. Describe the growth of cartilage.
3. Describe the comparative features of three types of cartilages.
4. Draw a neat labeled diagram of elastic cartilage.
5. Draw a neat labeled diagram of white fibro-cartilage.

Chapter 8

BONE/SCLEROUS TISSUE

Objectives

1. The knowledge of structure and functions of bones is necessary to understand the various types of fractures and pathological conditions.

2. The growth and blood supply of bones is necessary for understanding the remodeling of bones.

3. The different type of bone cells and their histological appearance is important to know the abnormal cells.

Definition: Bones are specialized dense connective tissue, made up of cells (osteocytes) and dense intercellular matrix with calcium salts and blood vessels. Total number of bones in humans is 206.

Functions of Bones

- Bones form the basic frame work of the body;
- Serve as levers for the muscles;
- Protect the underlying viscera;
- Contain bone-marrow thus helping in the formation of RBCs;
- Storehouse of calcium and phosphorus.

Gross Structure of Bones

- Bone consists of outer layer called as **compact** layer and an inner layer called as **cancellous/spongy** layer.

- Each bone is covered by periosteum (there's no periosteum in sesamoid bones), inner medullary cavity is filled with bone marrow, lined by inner vascular membrane called as endosteum.

- Periosteum has an outer fibrous layer (collagen) and an inner cellular layer and vascular layer called as osteogenic layer (immature osteoblasts).

Functions of Periosteum

+ Protects the bone, gives attachment to muscles and ligaments;

+ Maintains the shape of the bone;

+ Provides nutrition through its periosteal vessels;

+ Helps in sub-periosteal deposits of bone formation, increasing the width of the bone.

Classification of Bones

1. **According to Position**

   Axial Bones: skull, vertebrae, ribs, sternum;

   Appendicular Bones

   + Upper limb bones: clavicle, scapula, humerus, etc.

   + Lower limb: hip bone, femur, tibia, etc.

2. **According to Ossification**

   + Membranous, cartilagenous and membrano-cartilagenous bones.

3. **According to Shape**

   + Long, short, flat, irregular, pneumatic, sesamoid and accessory bones.

Parts of a Long Bone

+ Epiphysis; diaphysis and metaphysis.

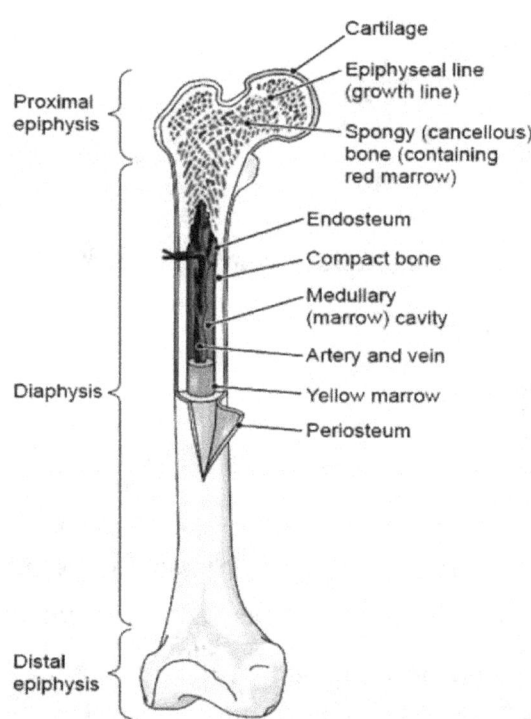

Parts of Long Bone: 1

1. **EPIPHYSIS:** The epiphysis ossifies from secondary centre; there are three types of epiphysis–

   ◆ **Pressure Epiphysis:** Transmits the body weight and protects the epiphyseal cartilage, e.g. heads of femur and humerus, condyles of femur and tibia.

   ◆ **Traction Epiphysis:** Produced by the pull of the muscles like tubercles of humerus and trochanters of femur.

   ◆ **Atavistic Epiphysis:** It's a phylogenetically independent bone attached to a host bone to receive the nutrition from it. It grows like a parasite, e.g. Coracoid process of scapula, posterior tubercle of talus (trigonum).

   ◆ **Aberrant:** Any additional epiphyseal centre seen in the distal end of first metacarpal is called as aberrant epiphysis, normally every metacarpal bone has only one epiphyseal centre at distal end except the first one which has epiphyseal centre at proximal end.

   The epiphysis unites with the diaphysis through the epiphyseal plate/hyaline cartilage.

   ◆ **Law of Union of Epiphysis:** The epiphyseal/secondary centre which appears first, unites last with the diaphysis and vice-versa (except fibula), this is also called as the growing end of the bone. The wrist and shoulder of upper limb and the knee of lower limb are the growing ends of the bones.

Parts of the Bone

2. **DIAPHYSIS:** This part of the bone ossifies from primary centre and forms the shaft of the bone.

3. **METAPHYSIS:** Ends of the diaphysis is called as metaphysis, wherein the bone grows in length. It is the most active growing area of a long bone. It is highly vascular with rich blood vessels in form of hair-pin like capillary loops, it is prone for infections. It gives attachment to muscles, ligaments and joint capsules.

Types of Long Bones

Typical; short long and modified.

   ◆ **Typical Long Bones:** Has 2 epiphyses and 1 diaphysis, e.g. limb bones-humerus, femur, etc.

   ◆ **Short Long Bones:** Has only 1 epiphysis at one end, e.g. metacarpals, metatarsals and phalanges, etc.

   ◆ **Modified Long Bones:** E.g. clavicle is the only long bone lying horizontally without the medullary cavity, ossifies in membrane. It is weight-bearing and transmits weight of upper limb to the axial bones. Vertebral body is another example.

   ◆ **Short Long Bones:** Carpal and tarsal bones have cubical shapes, they ossify in cartilage after birth, except talus, calcaneus and cuboid bones, which ossify at intra-uterine life itself.

- **Flat Bones:** There are two tables of compact bones with the spongy bone in the centre. E.g. Scapula, vault of skull, sternum, ribs, and etc. The spongy bone/diploe contains numerous veins.
- **Irregular Bones:** Bones of base of skull, vertebrae, hip bone, etc.

Pneumatic Bones

These contain air-filled spaces lined by mucous membrane, lying close to nasal cavity, e.g. maxilla, ethmoid bones, this makes the bones lighter; helps in resonance of vibrations of sound; acts as an air-conditioning chambers by adding humidity and temperature to the inspired air.

Sesamoid Bones (sesame = seed)

These bones develop within the tendons of the muscles; they act as pulleys for muscular contraction, e.g. pisiform in the tendon of flexor carpi ulnaris muscle, patella in quadriceps femoris, flabella in lateral head of Gastrocnemius, etc.

Its peculiarities include, they develop in tendons, ossify after birth, devoid of periosteum and absence of Haversian canals. They act as pulleys during muscle contraction.

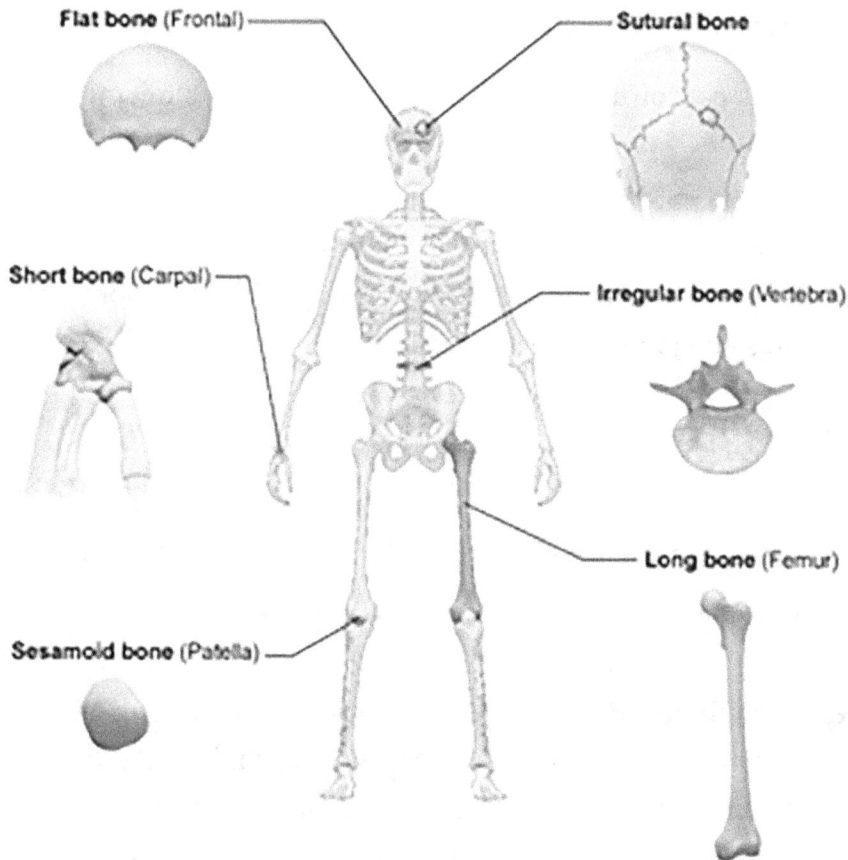

Classification of Bones by Shape

Types of Bones: 2

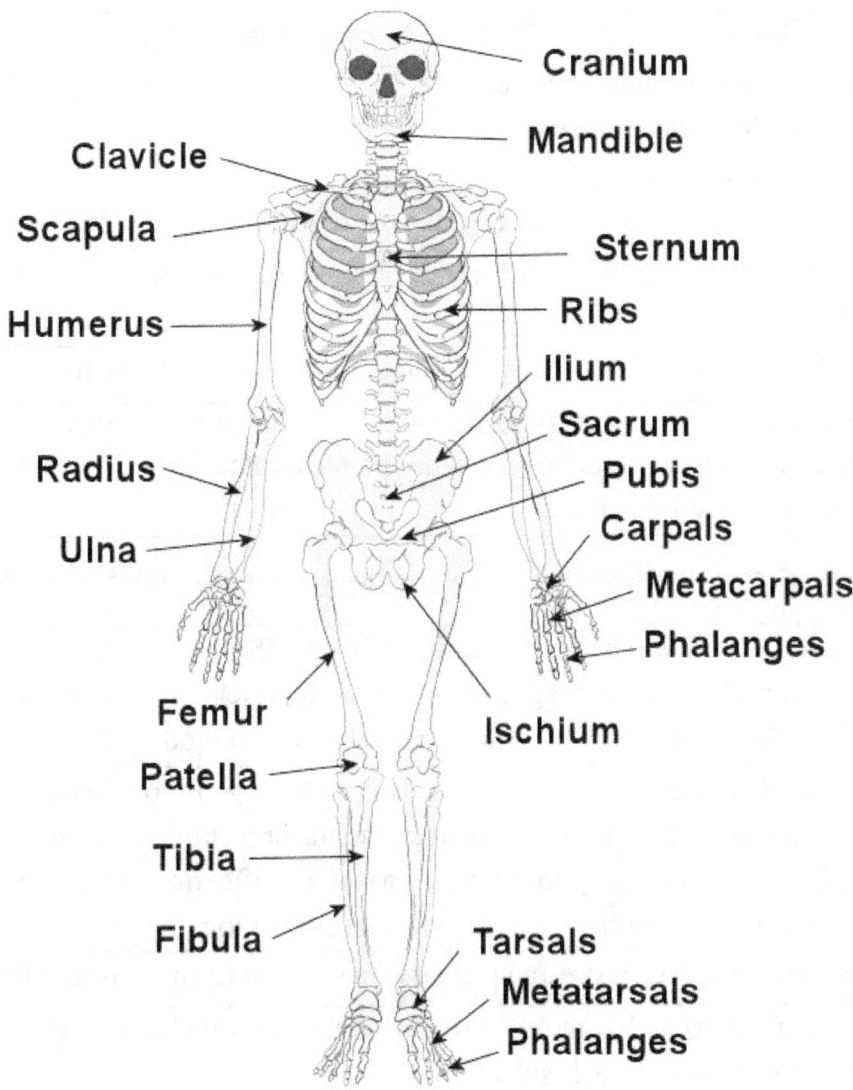

Human Skeletal Bones: 3

Laws of Ossification

♦ The point where the ossification begins is known as Primary ossification centre, which appear before birth except cuneiform, navicular bones.

♦ Secondary centres appear after birth, except lower end of femur.

♦ Ossification centre appears near to the growing end of the long bones.

♦ The epiphysis that that ossifies first fuses with the shaft last, except lower end of fibula.

♦ The epiphysis towards which nutrient artery is directed unites with the shaft last.

Ossification of Bone

♦ The process of formation of bone is called as **ossification,** wherein the osteoblasts undergo differentiation and secrete organic intercellular substance and collagen fibres, after this process there's deposition of calcium phosphate and this is known as *"calcification."*

STAGE 1	**MEMBRANOUS OSSIFICATION: E.g. Vault/skull bones.** **Mesenchymal cells differentiate into osteoblasts forming the centres of ossification, the collagen fibres appear.**
STAGE 2	Osteoblasts secrete organic intercellular substance; the cells show lacunae around them, cells keep proliferating by mitosis in a radiating manner forming trabeculae.
STAGE 3	Trabeculae join to form the cancellous bone, and the spaces in the trabeculae contain capillaries.
STAGE 4	Osteoblasts secrete alkaline phosphatase which calcifies the matrix.
STAGE 5	New bone is added to the ends of the trabeculae which increases the length of the bone, new bone at the sides of the trabeculae form the lamellae. Thus, new compact bone is formed.

There are **two types of ossifications:** membranous and cartilaginous ossifications.

STAGE 1	**CARTILAGINOUS/ENDOCHONDRAL OSSIFICATION: The mesenchymal cells form hyaline cartilaginous model with perichondrium, it grows in length by interstitial method and width by appositional method.**
STAGE 2	**Zone of proliferation:** cartilaginous cells arrange in longitudinal manner; **Zone of maturation:** Mature cells secrete chondroitin sulphate; **Zone of hypertrophy:** cells secrete alkaline phosphate; **Zone of calcification:** Calcium deposits in the matrix, cells die in-between due to lack of nutrition.
STAGE 3	Hypertrophied cells die and primary areolae are formed around them.
STAGE 4	Periosteal bud with osteoblasts are formed along with blood vessels, this bud forms the primary centre of ossification.

STAGE 1	**CARTILAGINOUS/ENDOCHONDRAL OSSIFICATION: The mesenchymal cells form hyaline cartilaginous model with perichondrium, it grows in length by interstitial method and width by appositional method.**
STAGE 2	**Zone of proliferation:** cartilaginous cells arrange in longitudinal manner; **Zone of maturation:** Mature cells secrete chondroitin sulphate; **Zone of hypertrophy:** cells secrete alkaline phosphate; **Zone of calcification:** Calcium deposits in the matrix, cells die in-between due to lack of nutrition.
STAGE 3	Hypertrophied cells die and primary areolae are formed around them.
STAGE 4	Periosteal bud with osteoblasts are formed along with blood vessels, this bud forms the primary centre of ossification.
STAGE 5	Osteoclasts destroys the calcified matrix to form the secondary areolae filled with marrow. Cells proliferate to form new cancellous bone.
STAGE 6	After birth the secondary ossification centre is formed, which goes to form the epiphysis.
STAGE 7	The epiphyseal cartilage is replaced by bone.

Blood Supply of Long Bones

Four sets of arteries supply the bone:

1. **Nutrient Artery:** It grows in the periosteal bud, enters the nutrient foramen in middle of the shaft, its highly tortuous, it divides into two branches, each branch again divides into small parallel vessels which run into metaphysis and form hair-pin like loops. These anastomose with other arteries around the metaphysis, which is the most vascular area, therefore, more prone for infections. The nutrient artery supplies the marrow and inner 2/3rd. of the compact bone.

2. **Juxta-Epiphyseal or Metaphyseal Arteries:** Small arteries from the joints run into the metaphysis and along the joint capsule.

3. **Epiphyseal Artery:** Supplies the epiphyseal cartilage and anastomose with the metaphyseal and nutrient arteries.

4. **Periosteal Artery:** Vessels enter the periosteum to enter the Volkmann's canals and supplies the Haversian system in the outer 1/3rd. of compact bone.

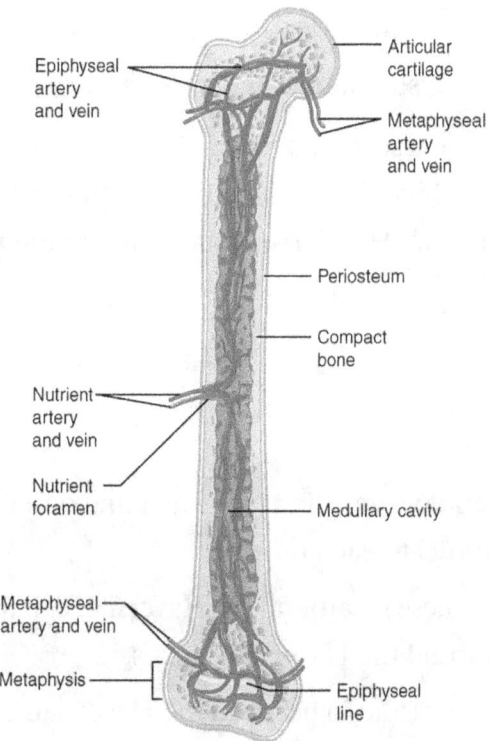

Blood Supply of Long Bone: 4

Growth of Bones

DIAPHYSIS: Length of the diaphysis increases by interstitial growth of cells of the epiphyseal cartilage, followed by deposition of bone at the metaphyseal end of diaphysis. Epiphyseal cartilage and metaphysis are the growing zones of the long bones. The epiphyseal cartilage shows the following zones of growth:

- Zone of resting cartilage;
- Zone of proliferating cells arranged in rows;
- Zone of mature cartilage secreting alkaline phosphatase;
- Zone of calcified cartilage.

EPIPHYSIS: Interstitial growth of articular cartilage helps the growth of epiphysis, both in width and length.

Factors affecting the bone growth:

- **Nutrition:** Vit. A, C and D are necessary for bone growth;
- **Hormones:** Growth hormone, parathormone and calcitonin are important for bone growth;
- Genetic factors;
- Mechanical factors.

Histology of Compact Bone

Compact bone is covered by periosteum, which has an outer fibrous layer and an inner cellular layer having osteoblasts. The endosteum lines the marrow cavity.

Transverse section/longitudinal section of bone: The central Haversian canal is surrounded by mature cells called osteocytes, which lie over thin bony plates called as lamellae, this constitutes the Haversian System/Osteon. The Haversian canals contain the blood vessels and nerve fibres for nutrition of the bone.

Types of Lamellae

There are three types:

1. **Circumferential Lamellae:** These lie at the inner and outer surface of the bones along the length of the bones parallel to each other.
2. **Concentric Lamellae:** These lie around the Haversian canals. The osteocytes are arranged in a circular manner around the Haversian canals.
3. **Interstitial Lamellae:** These lie in between the Haversian systems at angular intervals.

The lamellae is made up of organic and inorganic matrix. The ground substance consists of organic matrix – collagen (type 1) fibres, glycosaminoglycans, proteoglycans, glycoproteins and water.

Inorganic matrix – calcium and phosphorus forms the hydoxy-apatite crystals, which form the lamellae. Mg, Cl, Na, Carbonate salts are also present.

Osteocytes are surrounded by space called as lacunae. Each Haversian canal is connected to another canal through Volkmann's canal, these are connecting channels supplying nutrition to the bone between the marrow cavity and the external surface of the bones. The canaliculi are cellular processes of the cells that connect the cells with the Haversial canals and Volkman's canals to transfer nutrients from one Haversian system to another.

Types of Bone Cells

1. **Osteocytes:** These are mature cells, each cell is surrounded by lacuna and shows cytoplasmic processes called as canaliculi. The canaliculi help in diffusion of nutrients from one cell to another. The osteocytes help to remove/deposit the matrix and calcium when required.

2. **Osteoblasts:** These are immature cells and resemble the fibroblasts, and are derived from the osteogenic cells. These cells lay down the matrix and collagen fibres, and are rich in alkaline phosphatase. They help in calcification of matrix.

3. **Osteoclasts:** These large cells are seen at the sites of bone resorption, multinucleated cells with cytoplasm rich in acid phosphatase. These are bone removing cells, and help in remodeling of the bones through demineralization and removal of matrix.

   They are found over the surfaces of the bones and occupy the pits called as resorption bays or Howship's lacunae.

4. **Osteoprogenitor Cells:** These are of mesenchymal origin, they get converted into osteoblasts when stimulated. They are numerous in the fetus. In adults they are seen over the surfaces of the bone.

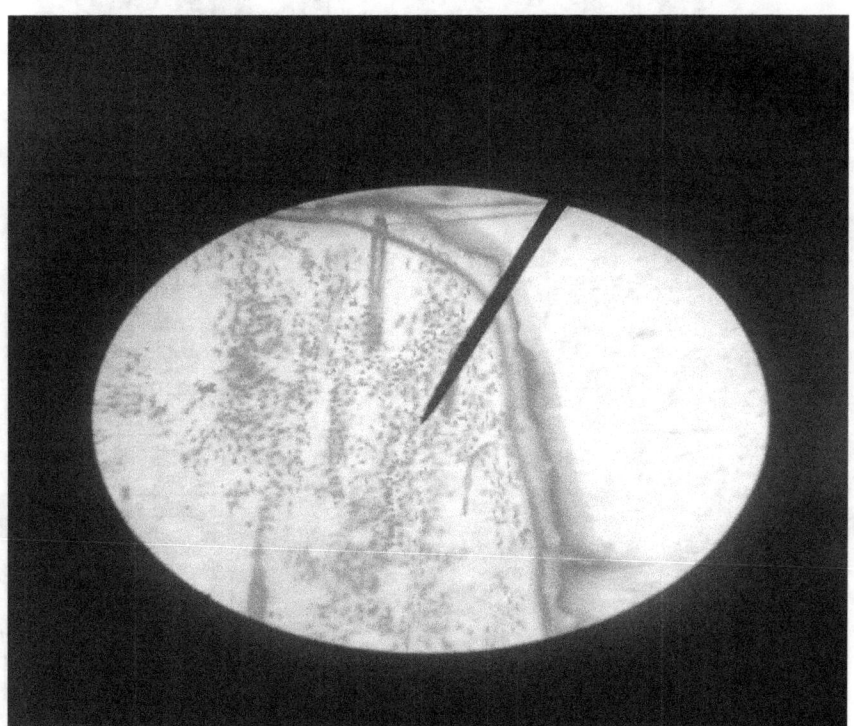

Longitudinal Section of Bone: 5

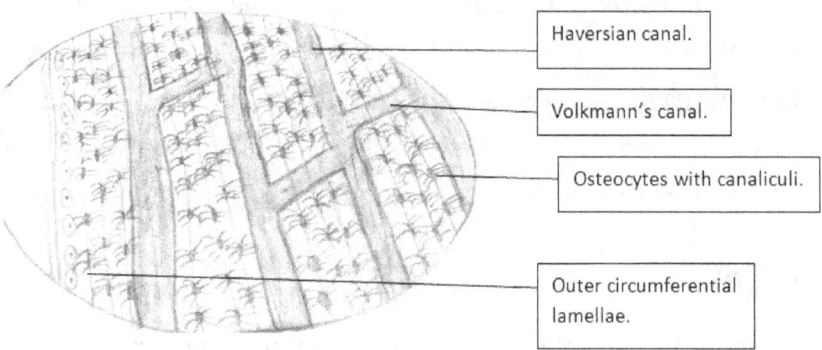

Haversian canal.

Volkmann's canal.

Osteocytes with canaliculi.

Outer circumferential lamellae.

Longitudinal Section of Bone: 6

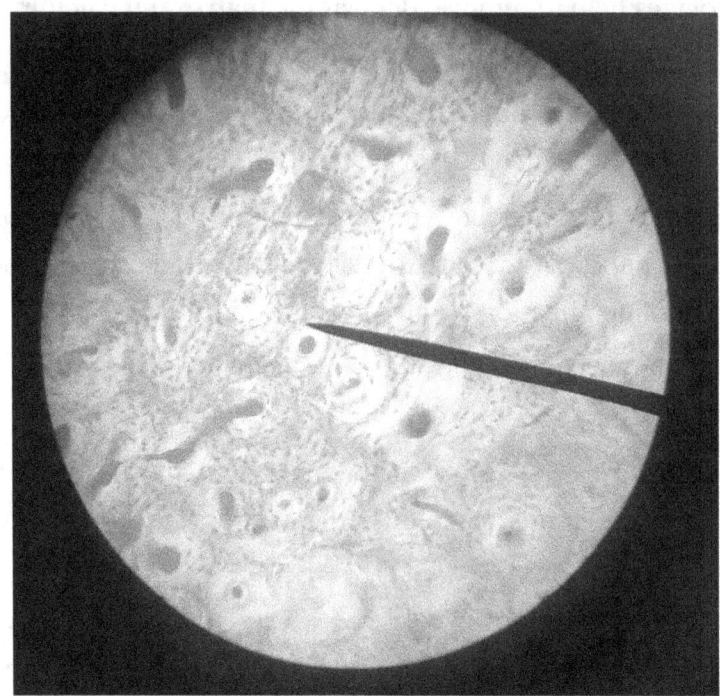

Transverse Section of Bone: 7

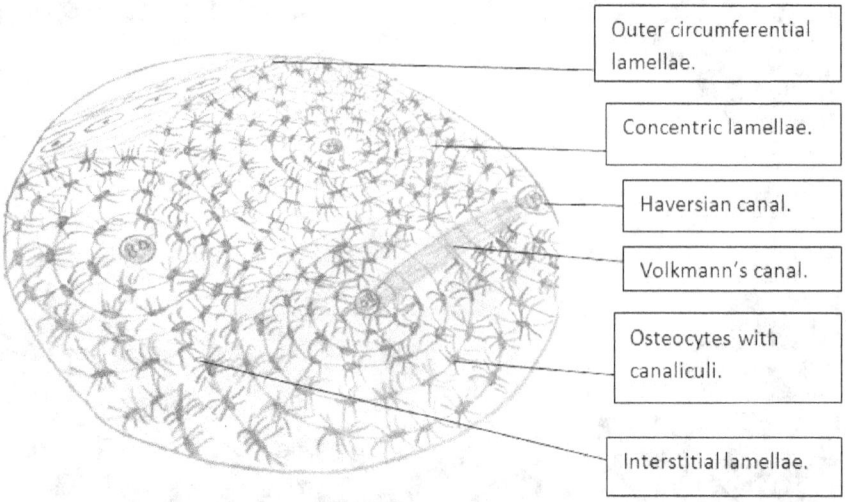

Outer circumferential lamellae.

Concentric lamellae.

Haversian canal.

Volkmann's canal.

Osteocytes with canaliculi.

Interstitial lamellae.

Transverse Section of Bone: 8

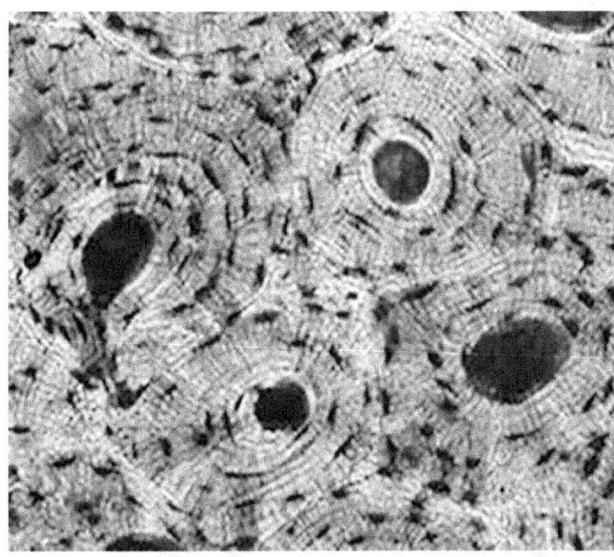

Transverse Section of Bone: 9

Applied Aspects

1. Any discontinuity in the bone is known as Fracture which is commonly due to trauma or injury. Incomplete breakage of bone is known as "hair-line fracture" or "Green stick fractures." Getting the two ends of the fractured bone fixed is called as "Fracture reduction." The new bone formation at the region of breakage is called as callus which later calcifies to form bone.

2. Osteoporosis is weakening of bones as seen in old age and due to hormonal imbalance especially in females, leading to easy breakage of bones.

Multiple Choice Questions

1. The bone cells that help in remodeling of bone is known as:

   a. Osteocytes;

   b. Osteoclasts;

   c. Osteoblasts;

   d. All of the above.

   (Answer: b)

2. All are the features of sesamoid bones except:

   a. They develop inside tendons,

   b. They do not have Haversian canal;

   c. They act as pulleys for muscle contraction;

   d. Vertebra is a good example.

   (Answer: d)

3. Examples of Pneumatic bones are the following except:

   a. Patella,

   b. Carpal bones;

   c. Facial bones;

   d. Tarsal bones.

   (Answer: c)

4. Example of Atavistic epiphysis is:

   a. Head of femur;

   b. Coracoid process of scapula;

   c. Tubercles of humerus;

   d. Trochanters of femur.

   (Answer: b)

5. Vertebrae are:

   a. Short long bones;

   b. Pneumatic bones;

   c. Irregular bones;

   d. Flat bones.

   (Answer: c)

Model Questions

Short Notes (5 Marks)

1. Classify bones giving examples for each.
2. Describe types of ossifications in detail.
3. Describe the Blood supply of long bones.

Short Answers (2 Marks)

1. Write the functions of bone.
2. Name the types of ossification.
3. Name the types of Epiphyses with examples.

Chapter 9

JOINTS (ARTHROLOGY)

Objectives

1. Study of joints known as Arthrology is very beneficial for medical students aspiring for Orthopedics.

2. Details of normal anatomy of various types of joints are important for identifying disorders of joints like: Osteoarthritis; Neuropathic joints as seen in leprosy, etc.

3. Dislocation of the joints can be reduced only when you know the normal relations of the joints.

Definition: A joint or articulation is a connection between two bones or more bones.

Classification

Can be classified in two ways:

1. Depending on nature of connecting medium;

2. Depending on the movements.

According to Connecting Media

1. Fibrous joints;

2. Cartilaginous joints;

3. Synovial joints.

1. **Fibrous Joints:** Connecting medium is fibrous tissue, immobile joint, its types are:

   a. Sutures;

   b. Gomphosis;

   c. Syndesmosis.

   a. **Sutures:** Seen in cranial bones, bones are joined together by sutural/fibrous ligament, after certain age it ossifies and the bones unite permanently by **Synostosis.**

   Types of Sutures: Sutura serrata, sutura denticulata, sutura plana, etc.

b.   **Gomphosis:** Articulation between a peg into a socket, like the tooth and the socket. The periodontal ligament binds the tooth to the bony socket.

c.   **Syndesmosis:** The inter-osseous membrane binds the bones together, e.g. tibio-fibular joint and radio-ulnar joint.

2.   **Cartilagenous Joints**: The articulation between the bones is by hyaline/fibro cartilage, they are slightly movable or immovable joints. There are two types:

a.   Synchondrosis/primary cartilaginous joints and

b.   Symphysis/secondary cartilaginous joints.

a.   **Synchondrosis:** The connecting medium is the hyaline cartilage which later undergoes ossification, they are immovable joints, e.g. between the epiphysis and diaphysis of a long bone.

b.   **Symphysis:** The bony surfaces are covered by hyaline cartilage, and the two bones are united by the white-fibro cartilage, they are slightly movable or immovable joints, e.g. pubic symphysis and inter-vertebral joints.

3.   **Synovial Joints:** These are highly movable joints, held together by the capsular ligament and lined by synovial membrane.

Characteristics of Synovial Joints

1.   Joint is surrounded by capsular ligament; and lined by synovial membrane;

2.   The ends of the bones are covered by articular cartilage;

3.   There's a space between the bony ends called as the joint cavity; which is filled with synovial fluid.

4.   The joint cavity contains articular discs/intra-articular cartilage/menisci.

5.   All the joints are highly movable joints.

Characteristic Features of Synovial Fluid

The synovial fluid is highly viscus/thick and is the dialysate of blood plasma containing **Hyaluronic acid**, which is secreted by the synovial cells and mast cells present in the synovial membrane. Hyaluronic acid causes the fluid to become viscus. The fluid contains WBC, macrophages, synovial cells.

Functions of Synovial Fluid

*   Maintains nutrition of cartilage;

*   Provides lubrication to the joint;

*   Lubrication provides smooth gliding movements of the joints;

- It prevents wear and tear of the articular cartilage covering the bony ends of the joint;
- Phagocytosis.

Classification of Synovial Joints

a. Depending on the articulating surfaces (simple/compound);

b. Depending on the axis of movement;

c. Depending on shape of articulating ends.

   a. Depending on the Articulating Surfaces: If there are only two articulating surfaces then it is called as simple, e.g. hip joint. If there are more than two surfaces then its called as compound, e.g. elbow joint.

   b. Depending on Axes of Movement:

   i. **Uni-Axial Joint:** The movement of the joint is around a single axis only e.g Elbow joint;

   ii. **Bi-Axial Joint:** The movement of the joint is at two axes e.g radio-carpal joint;

   iii. **Multi-Axial Joint:** There are three degree of movements, e.g. shoulder joint.

   c. Depending on the Shape of the Articulating Surfaces:

   - **Ball and Socket Joint:** Multi-axial joints, e.g. shoulder joint and hip joint.
   - **Condylar Joint:** Uni-axial joints, e.g. Temporomandibular/knee joints.
   - **Ellipsoid/Condyloid Joints:** Bi-axial joints, e.g. metacarpo-phalangeal joints.
   - **Saddle Joint:** Bi-axial joints, e.g. thumb joint.
   - **Hinge Joint:** Uni-axial joint, e.g. elbow/inter-phalangeal joints.
   - **Pivot Joint:** Uni-axial and rotation, e.g. atlanto-axial joint.
   - **Plane Joint:** Gliding movement, e.g. inter-carpal joints.

     1. **Depending on Movements:**

        - **Synarthrosis:** Immovable joints, e.g. skull bones;
        - **Amphiarthrosis:** Slightly movable joints, e.g. Pubic symphysis.
        - **Diarthrosis:** Freely movable joints, e.g. synovial joints.

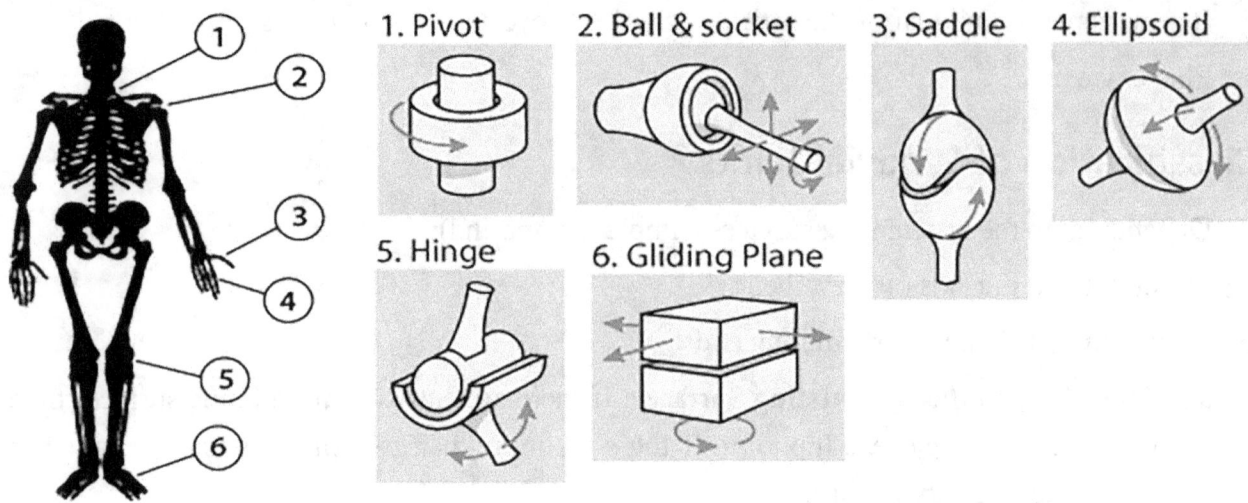

Types of Joints: 1

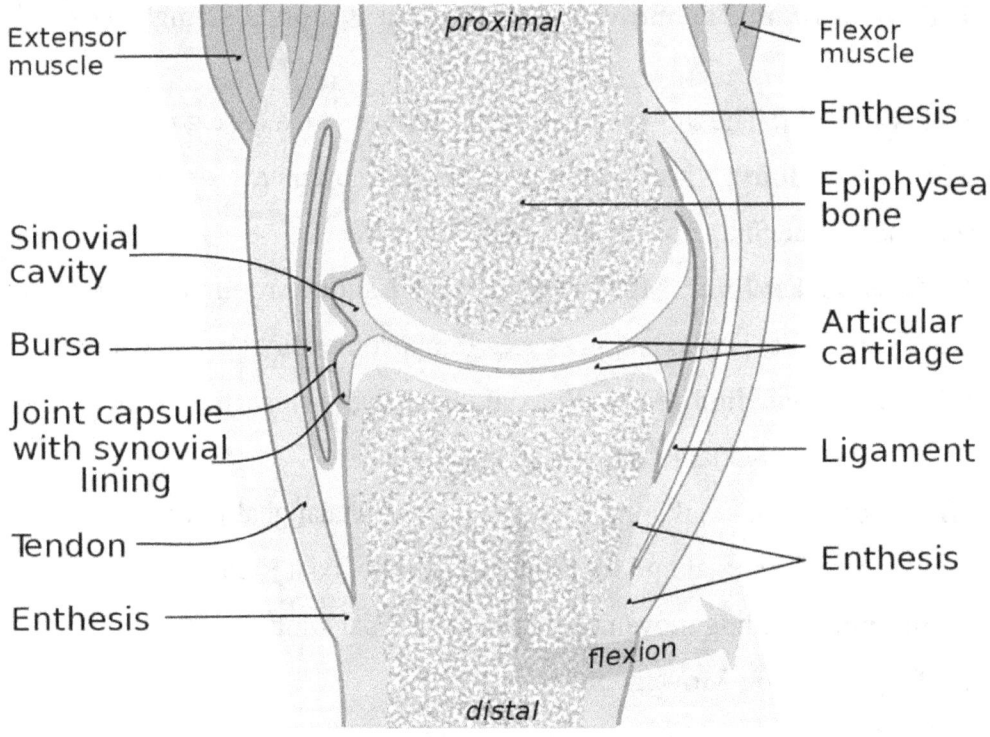

Synovial Joint: 2

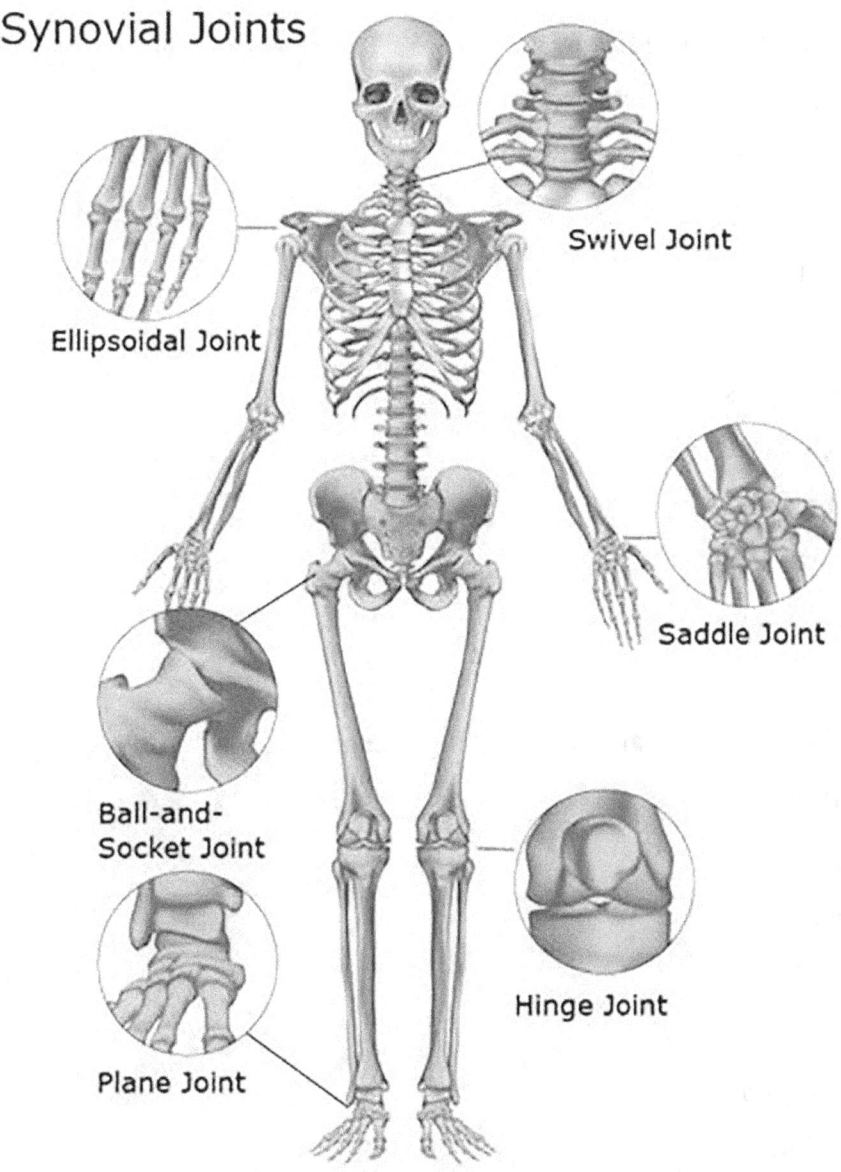

Synovial Joints

Ellipsoidal Joint

Swivel Joint

Saddle Joint

Ball-and-
Socket Joint

Hinge Joint

Plane Joint

Types of Synovial Joints: 3

Applied Aspects

1. Dislocations are very common especially in children and sports persons.

2. Ligamentous tears are common, leading to Sprain and are very painful.

3. Swelling and inflammation of synovial joint may be due to various pathological conditions like Rheumatoid arthritis, Neuropathic joint, Osteoarthritis, etc.

Multiple Choice Questions

1. Example of Pivot type of joint is:
   a. Atlanto-axial type of joint;
   b. Inter-vertebral joint;
   c. Inter-carpal joint;
   d. Pubic symphysis.
   (Answer: a)

2. Articular cartilage is:
   a. Hyaline cartilage;
   b. White fibro cartilage;
   c. Elastic cartilage;
   d. Yellow cartilage.
   (Answer: b)

3. Features of Synovial fluid are the following except:
   a. Lubrication;
   b. Phagocytosis;
   c. Nutrition;
   d. Binds the bones.
   (Answer: d)

4. Saddle type of joint is:
   a. Thumb joint;
   b. Shoulder joint;
   c. Hip joint;
   d. Elbow joint.
   (Answer: a)

Model Questions

Short Notes (5 Marks)

1. Classify Synovial joints with examples.
2. Write salient features of Synovial joints.
3. Classify Joints giving examples for each.

Chapter 10

MUSCULAR TISSUE

Objectives

1. Classification of muscle is important to understand the range of movement and force of contraction.
2. The study of normal microscopic structure of different types of muscles is important for surgeons.
3. You need to know the normal structure of Neuromuscular junction in order to understand its Physiology.

Definition: Contractile tissue of the body derived from embryonic mesoderm/mesenchyme, brings about movement of organs & body.

Musculus = mouse

Exceptions – arrector pilorum, muscle of iris & myoepithelial cells of glands, derived from ectoderm.

Classification of Muscular Tissues

Three types:

- Skeletal muscle/voluntary/striped muscle;
- Cardiac muscle/involuntary/striped muscle;
- Smooth muscle/involuntary/unstriped muscle.

Differences between the three types of muscles are shown in the following table:

Features	Skeletal Muscle	Cardiac Muscle	Smooth Muscle
Control	Voluntary	Involuntary	Involuntary
Histology	Striped	Striped	Unstriped
Location	Skeleton	Heart (Myocardium)	Git, Rt, Ugt.

(Contd.)

Muscle Fibres	Unbranched, multi-nucleated, peripherally placed, cross-striations	Branched, uni-nucleated, centrally-placed, faint cross-striations, inter-calated discs.	Unbranched, spindle shaped, uni-nucleated, centrally placed, no cross-striations.
Rhythmicity	Absent	Present	Present
Nerve supply	Somatic	Autonomic	Autonomic
Stretch receptors	Present	Absent	Absent
Neuromuscular junction	Present	Absent	Absent
Syncytium	True syncytium	Not true syncytium	-------

Other Contractile Units

* **Myoepithelial Cells** – flat cells present in glands of lacrimal, salivary and mammary, expels the secretions from cells.

* **Myofibroblasts** – seen in wound healing process.

* **Properties Shared by Three Muscles** – Irritability (sensitive to stimuli), contractility, extensibility and elasticity.

Skeletal Muscle/Voluntary Muscle

Skeletal muscles are attached to skeleton & function as levers to move the body.

Functions

* Locomotion: e.g. walking,

* Heat production: metabolism in cells produces heat e.g. exercises,

* Maintains body posture;

* Provides body support;

* Muscles (deltoid) are used for giving intra muscular injections.

Histology

Each muscle consists of muscle fibres – myofibrils – myofilaments (actin & myosin).

Each muscle is covered by C.T. – Epimysium,

Each muscle fibre bundle – Perimysium,

Each muscle fibre – Endomysium.

Each myocyte is covered by sarcolemma, & the cytoplasm is called sarcoplasm. The cross-striations are due to dark and light bands in the cytoplasm.

Under the polarized light: dark band (A-band) anisotropic and light band (I-band) isotropic. Middle of dark band is a light line – H-line, a dark line in this zone is M-line.

Middle of light band is a dark line – Z-line.

The region between two Z-lines is called as sarcomere – contractile unit of a myofibril.

Depending on colour; direction of muscle fibres; force of action and action of muscles.

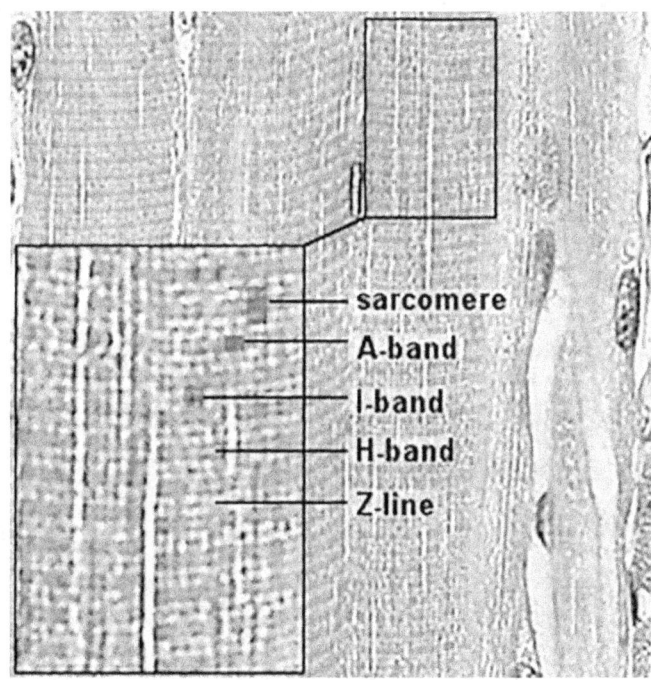

Skeletal Muscle: 1

Striated (Skeletal) Muscle

Striations of Skeletal Muscle: 2

Skeletal Muscle: 3 (for figure refer page no. 74)

Skeletal Muscle: 4 (for figure refer page no. 75)

Cardiac Muscle: 5 (for figure refer page no. 75)

Cardiac Muscle: 6 (for figure refer page no. 76)

Classification of Voluntary Muscles

♦ **According to colour** (amount of Myo-Hemoglobin) – Red and white muscles.

According to the Direction of Muscle Fibres

♦ **Parallel Muscle Fibres:** Platysmus

♦ **Strap Muscles:** Sartorius, Rectus abdominis.

♦ **Quadrate:** Quadratus lumborum.

♦ **Fusiform:** Biceps.

♦ **Pennate Muscles:** Fibres run obliquely

    a. Unipennate – Flexor Pollicis Longus, Extensor Digitorum Longus.

    b. Bipennate – Rectus femoris, Dorsal Interosseous muscles of hand.

    c. Multipennate – Deltoid muscle.

    d. Circumpennate – Tibialis anterior muscle,

♦ **Spiral Muscle:** Pectoralis Major, Supinator,

♦ **Cruciate Muscle:** Masseter, Sternocleidomastoid muscle,

♦ **Sphincteric Muscles:** Orbicularis Oris.

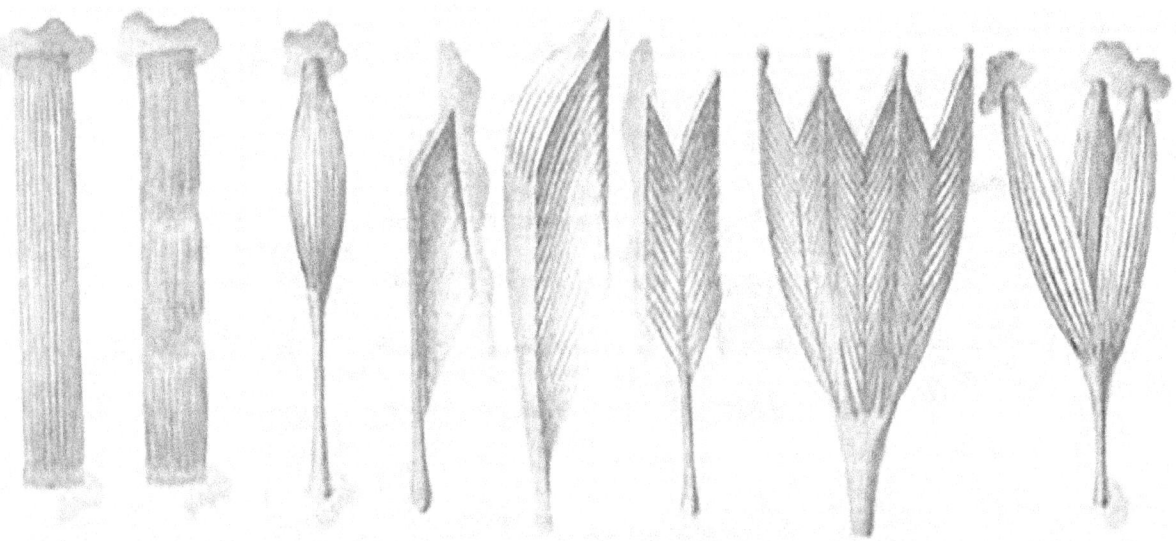

Types of Muscles Depending on Direction of Fibres: 7

Depending on Force of Action

When swing component (angular movement of a joint) is powerful it's called as a spurt muscles (Brachialis), if there's powerful shunt component (muscle draws the bone towards a joint) then it's called as shunt muscle (Brachioradialis).

Depending on Action of Muscle

- **Agonists:** group of muscles which bring about movement along the line of gravity, reverse of this is called Paradoxical contraction.
- **Antagonists:** group of muscles that oppose the desired movement and relax the prime movers (law of reciprocal innervations).
- **Fixation Muscles:** group of muscles that stabilize the proximal joints and allow movements at distal joints by the prime movers.
- **Synergists:** special fixation muscles, which cross two or more joints and prevent undesired movement at intermediate joints.

Depending on Shape/Size/Heads/Actions

- Site – Pectus = chest, Pectoralis major muscle,
- Shape – Trapezius (trapezoid in shape),
- Action – Extensor Carpi Ulnaris, Flexor Carpi Radialis,
- Heads – Biceps (2 heads), triceps (3 heads), quadriceps (4 heads),
- Size – gluteus maximus (huge muscle), gluteus medius (medium sized muscle), gluteus minimus (small sized muscle).

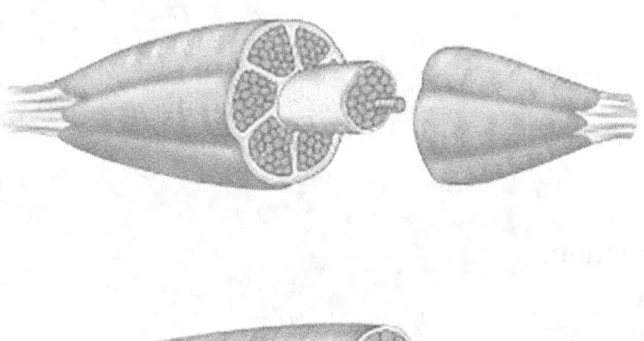

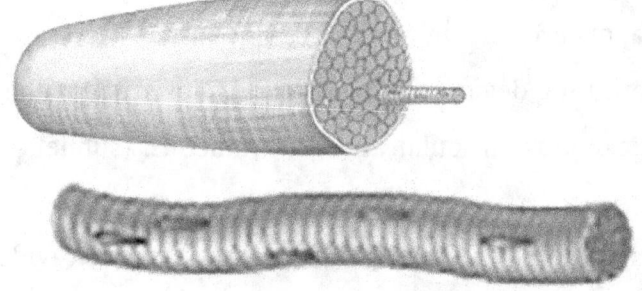

Coverings of Muscle Bundle: 8

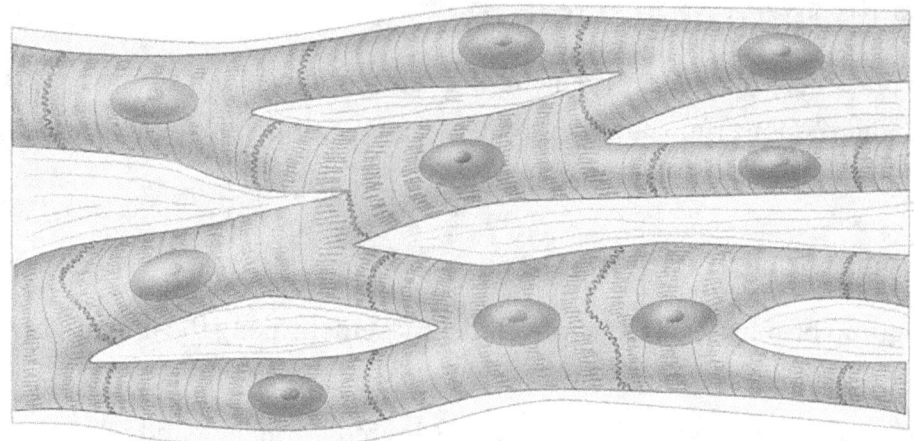

Cardiac Muscle: 9

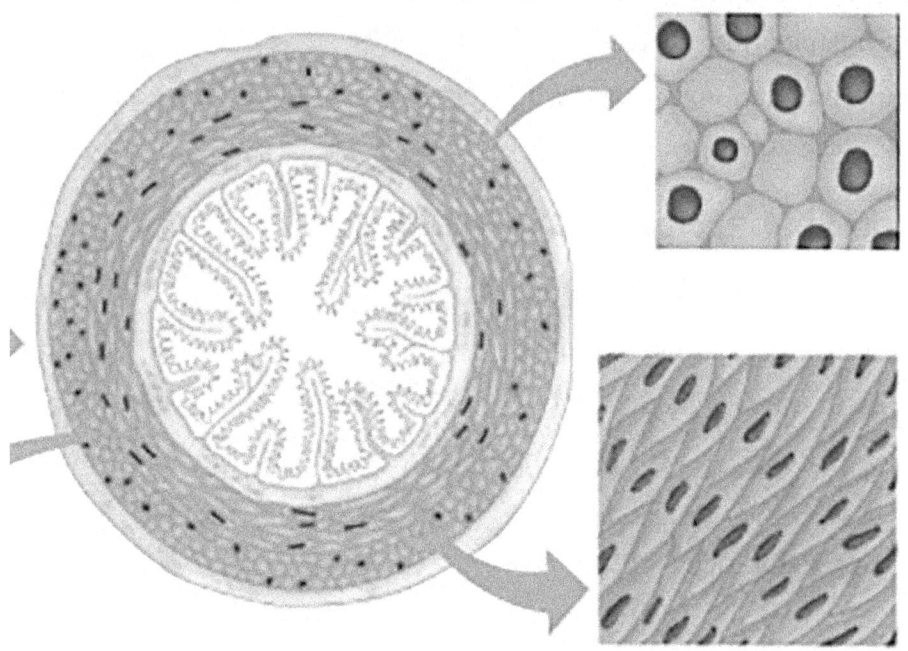

Smooth Muscle: 10

Parts of a Muscle

- Tendon at point of insertion,
- Muscle belly,
- Origin: from bone/aponeurosis/tendons/subcutaneous,
- Synovial bursa – lubricating device, reduces friction, closed sac with synovial fluid.

Types of Bursas: Subtendinous, articular and subcutaneous. (subdeltoid/subacromial bursa is largest).

Blood Supply: The arteries ramify into the epi and perimysium and divide into capillaries to enter the endomysium.

Nerve Supply: 60% motor (through alpha and gamma neurons) and 40% sensory (free nerve endings, golgi tendon organs and muscle spindles – sensory receptor organs which maintain the muscle tone.

- **Motor Point:** Is the point of entry of a nerve trunk into the muscle, into deep parts.
- **Motor Unit:** A single motor neuron suppling a group of muscle fibres e.g. extra-ocular muscles.

Neuromuscular Junction: Is the junction between the terminal end of axon (motor end plate) and sarcolemma of a muscle fibre (sole plate). The motor end plate contains synaptic vesicles with neurotransmitters (Ach).

Applied Anatomy

- Loss of motor power to produce movement is called paralysis (hemiplegia/polio).
- Loss of movement for a long time as seen in hemiplegia causes muscular atrophy.
- **Myasthenia Gravis:** It's a auto-immune disease where body produces antibodies against the body through Ach receptors at neuro-muscular junction, leading to flaccid paralysis.
- **Rigor Mortis:** A state of temporary rigidity developing in the muscles after death.
- Tetanus and rabies produces muscular rigidity.
- Sarcoma is tumour of muscle.
- The small bursae which are fluid filled closed sacs lying beneath the tendons can get infected leading to bursitis.

Multiple Choice Questions

1. Intercalated disc is seen in:
   a. Cardiac muscle;
   b. Skeletal muscle;
   c. Smooth muscle;
   d. Strap muscle.
   (Answer: a)

2. Example of multi-pennate muscle is:
   a. Lumbricals;
   b. Biceps;
   c. Deltoid;
   d. Palmaris longus.
   (Answer: c)

3. The True syncytium is:

    a. Cardiac muscle;

    b. Skeletal muscle;

    c. Smooth muscle;

    d. None of the above.

    (Answer: b)

4. One of the following disease is related to muscle rigidity:

    a. Typhoid;

    b. Malaria;

    c. Tetanus;

    d. Myasthenia Gravis.

    (Answer: c)

Model Questions

Write Short Notes On (5 Marks)

1. Microscopic picture of Cardiac muscle.

2. Histology of Skeletal muscle.

3. Classify Muscles giving examples for each.

Short Answers (2 Marks)

1. Write differences between cardiac and skeletal muscles.

2. Draw a neat labeled diagram of cardiac/skeletal muscle.

Chapter 11

BLOOD VASCULAR SYSTEM

Objectives

1. The sound knowledge of the vascular system is important to understand cardio-vascular emergencies like vascular occlusions like Atherosclerosis causing Myocardial infarction.

2. The microscopic picture of the normal vessels helps us to understand the pathogenesis of atherosclerotic plaques.

Definition: The **arteries** carry oxygenated blood from the heart to the tissues, they are tubular structures, which branch repeatedly to supply various organs. The **veins** carry deoxygenated blood from the tissues to the lungs for oxygenation.

Large arteries (elastic arteries) arise from the aorta to branch into **medium sized arteries (muscular arteries)**, which divide into **arterioles,** these divide into tiny **capillaries/sinusoids,** the exchange of nutrients and oxygen takes place through these capillaries. Blood from capillaries goes to the **venules (small veins)**, these venules join to form the **veins,** the blood from here goes to the IVC and SVC to reach the heart. About 5 liters of blood circulates in the vascular system.

Functions of Arteries

1. Arteries conduct and distribute **oxygenated blood** to the tissues.

2. They help to maintain **continuous blood flow.**

3. Arterioles regulate the **blood pressure.**

4. **Arterial anastomosis** provides alternate route for blood in case of compression/blockage of arteries, this is called as collateral circulation.

5. **End arteries** do not anastomose with other arteries, therefore, the tissues it supplies dies due to lack of blood supply, e.g. central artery of retina, mesenteric arteries of intestines (vasa recta), arteries of spleen, kidney and lung.

6. **Arterio-venous anastomosis/shunt** helps to regulate the body temperature.

Types of Arteries

1. Large sized artery/elastic artery, e.g. aorta;

2. Medium sized artery/muscular artery, e.g. radial/brachial arteries;

3. Arterioles, capillaries and sinusoids.

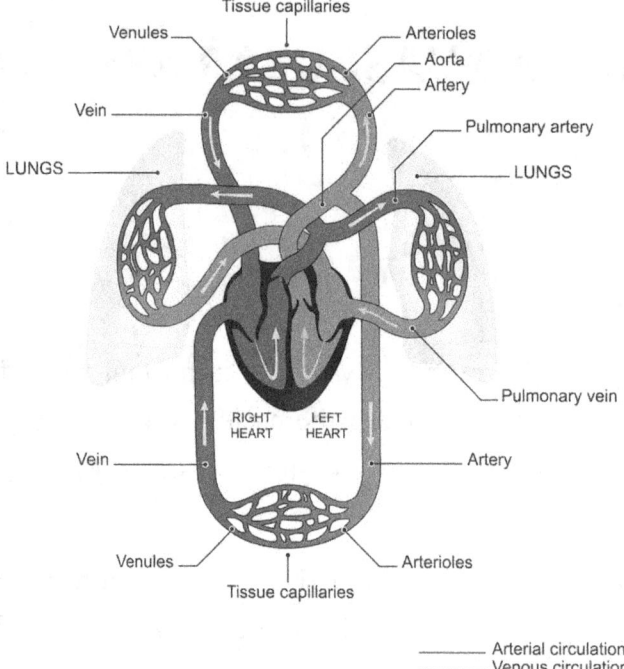

Blood Vascular System: 1

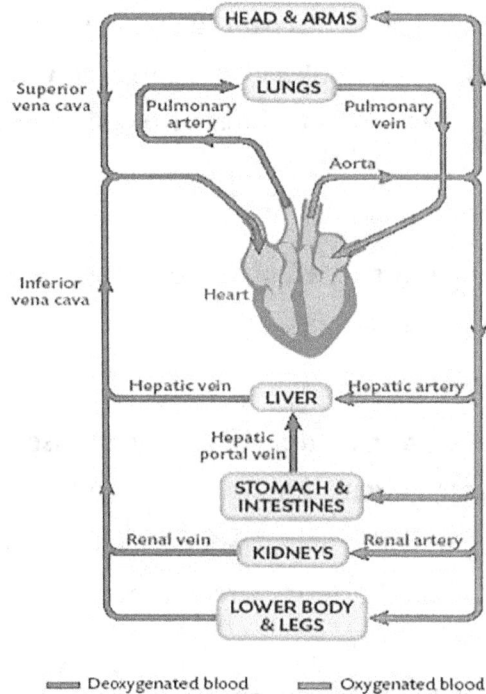

Blood Vascular System: 2

Histology of Large Sized Artery (Elastic Artery) and Medium Sized Artery (Muscular Arteries)

All the arteries have the following three layers/tunics:

a. Tunica intima;

b. Tunica media and

c. Tunica adventitia.

   a. **Tunica Intima:** Has flat endothelial cells lying over a basement membrane and lining the inner wall of the artery. These endothelial cells are supported by an elastic layer called as internal elastic lamina.

   b. **Tunica Media:** It is a thick layer, made up of smooth muscle cells and plenty of elastic fibres. The smooth muscle cells are more in muscular artery whereas, the elastic fibres are more in large sized artery. Large sized arteries include: Aorta, pulmonary trunk, etc. Medium sized arteries are Radial artery, Brachial artery, etc.

   c. **Tunica Adventitia:** It consists of loose connective tissue with elastic and collagen fibres. It contains small arterioles called as **vasa vasorum** which supplies nutrition to the outer aspect of the arterial wall especially in large sized arteries, inner wall is supplied by direct diffusion.

Large Sized Artery: 3 (for figure refer page no. 76)

Medium Sized Artery: 4 (for figure refer page no. 77)

Histology of Veins

♦ It consists of three coats as the artery.

♦ Tunica intima has endothelial cells. The wall is very thin and the lumen is collapsed.

♦ The internal elastic lamina is absent.

♦ Tunica media is thin and consists of elastic fibres, smooth muscle cells and numerous collagen fibres.

♦ Tunica adventitia is more, made up of elastic fibres and smooth muscle cells.

Examples of large sized veins are SVC, IVC.

Large Sized Vein: 5 (for figure refer page no. 77)

Large Sized Artery: 6 (for figure refer page no. 78)

Medium Sized Artery: 7 (for figure refer page no. 78)

Large Sized Vein: 8 (for figure refer page no. 79)

CAPILLARIES: These are lined by thin endothelial cells; the pericytes/contractile cells are seen in the basal lamina. They do not have tunica media and tunica adventitia. There are two types of capillaries:

1. **Continuous Capillaries**: Are seen in muscles, brain, skin, etc. There is no gap in the endothelial cell.

2. **Fenestrated Capillaries:** There are gaps in-between the endothelial cells, e.g. pancreas, endocrine glands, renal- glomeruli, intestinal villi, etc.

SINUSOIDS: These are large, irregular, lined by endothelial cells with large pores for diffusion of blood and tissue fluids. Sinusoids are found in bone-marrow, spleen, parathyroid gland and adrenal gland.

Applied Aspects

1. The study of coronary arteries and site of occlusion due to atherosclerosis can be determined by imaging technique like Angiography.

2. Normal Blood pressure is 120/80 mmHg.

3. Vascular accidents can be due to Thrombosis, Embolism and Haemorrhage.

Multiple Choice Questions

1. In Large sized artery the tunica media contains numerous:
   a. Muscular fibres;
   b. Elastic fibres;
   c. Collagen fibres;
   d. Reticular fibres.
   (Answer: b)

2. Example of large sized vein is:
   a. Cephalic vein;
   b. Median cubital vein,
   c. Inferior venacava;
   d. Basilic vein.
   (Answer: c)

3. The tunica adventitia is comparatively more in:

    a. Arteries;

    b. Veins;

    c. Capillaries;

    d. Sinusoids.

    (Answer: b)

Model Questions

Write Short Notes On (5 Marks)

1. Histology of Large sized artery with the help of neat labeled diagram.

2. Microscopic picture of large sized Vein.

3. Microscopic structure of Medium sized artery.

Short Answers (2 Marks)

1. Write any three differences between microscopic structure of artery and vein.

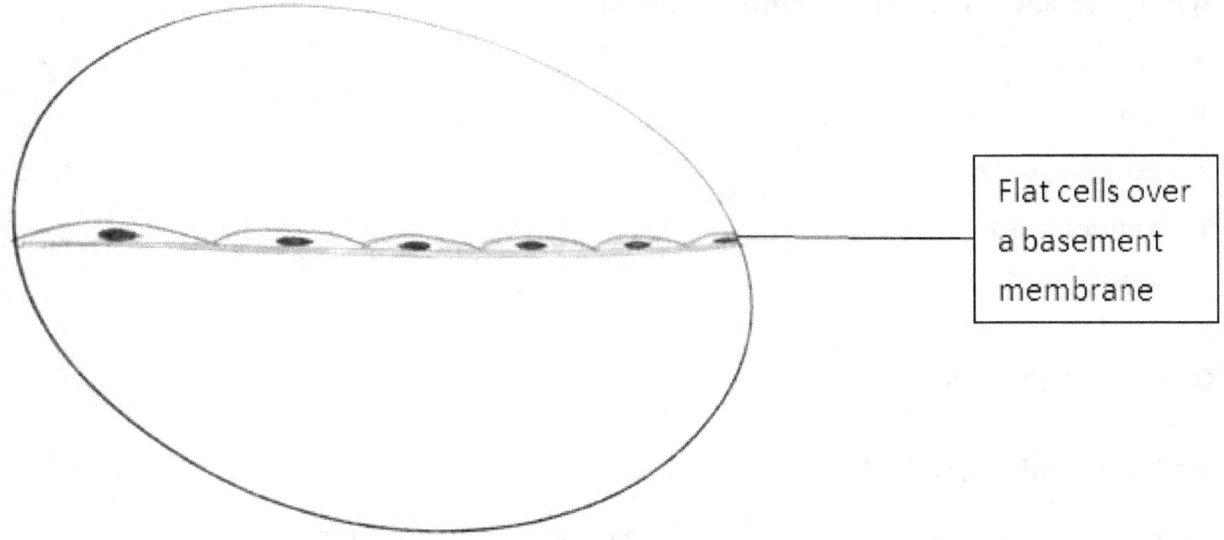

Flat cells over a basement membrane

Simple Squamous Epithelium: 1

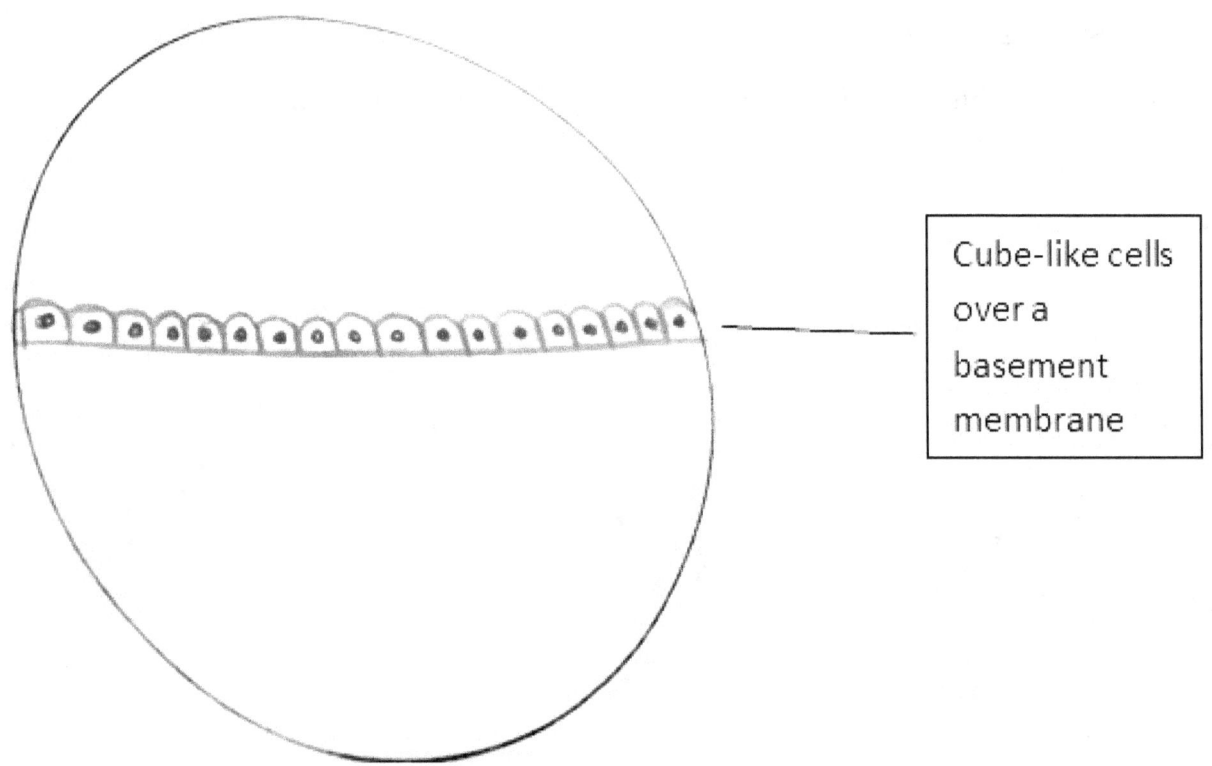

Cube-like cells over a basement membrane

Simple Cuboidal Epithelium: 2

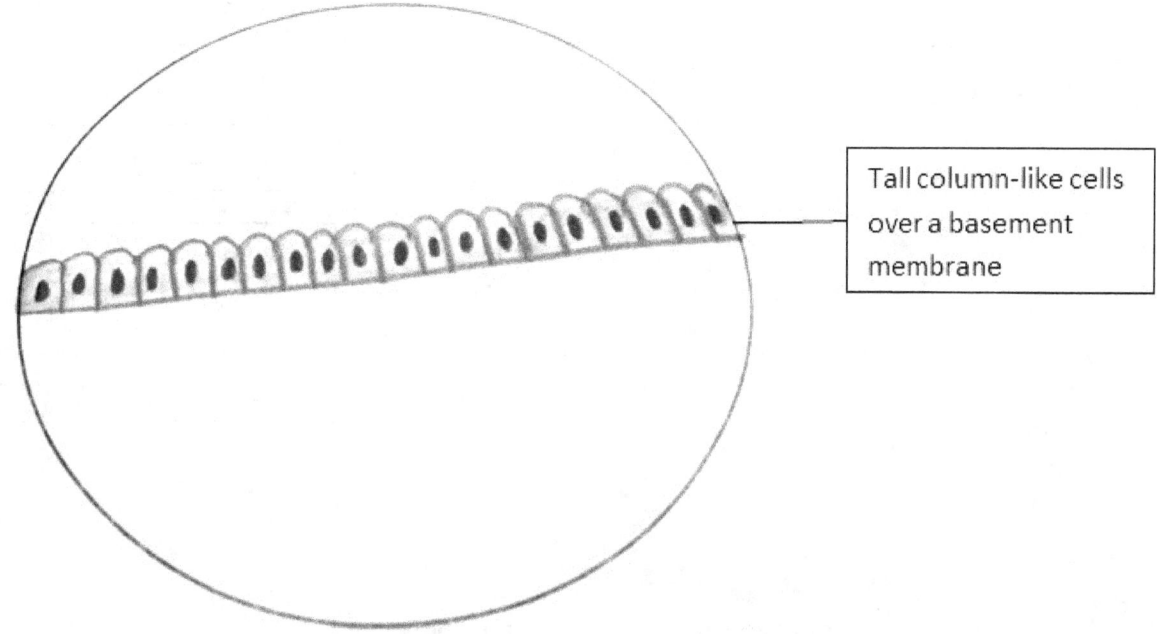

Tall column-like cells over a basement membrane

Simple Columnar Epithelium: 3

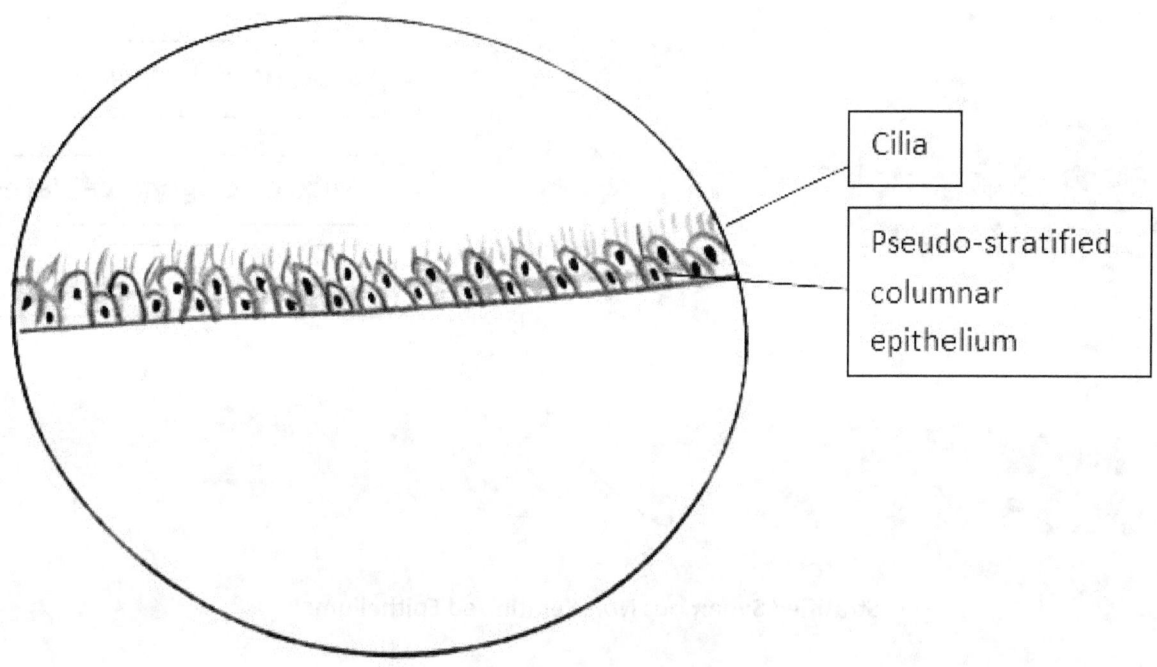

Cilia

Pseudo-stratified columnar epithelium

Pseudostratified Epithelium: 4

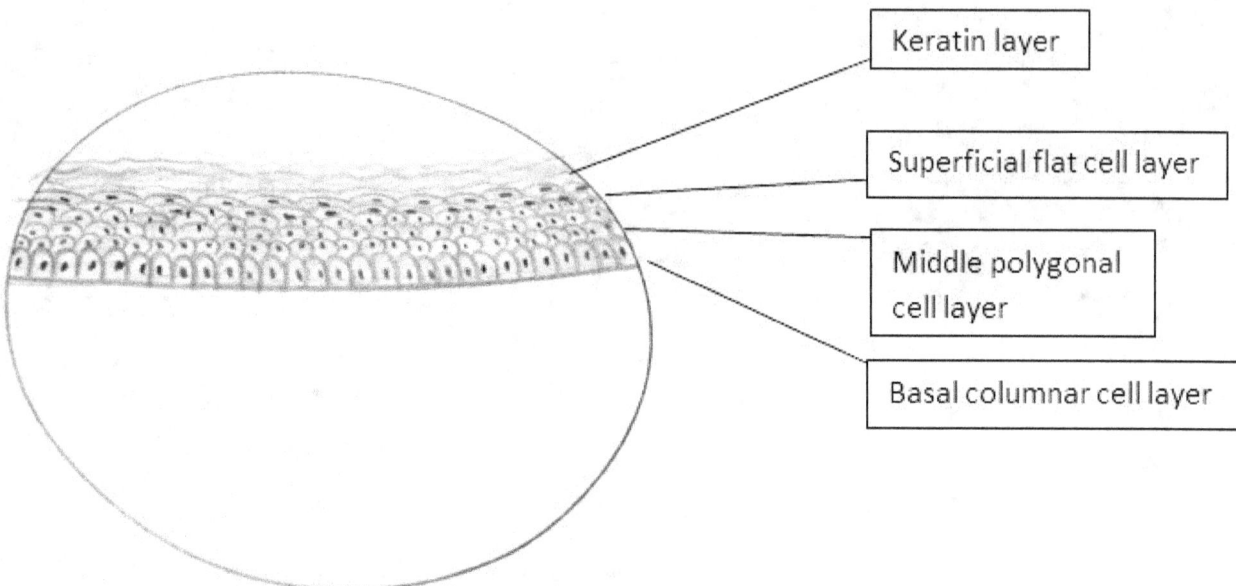

Keratin layer

Superficial flat cell layer

Middle polygonal cell layer

Basal columnar cell layer

Stratified Squamous Keratinized Epithelium: 7

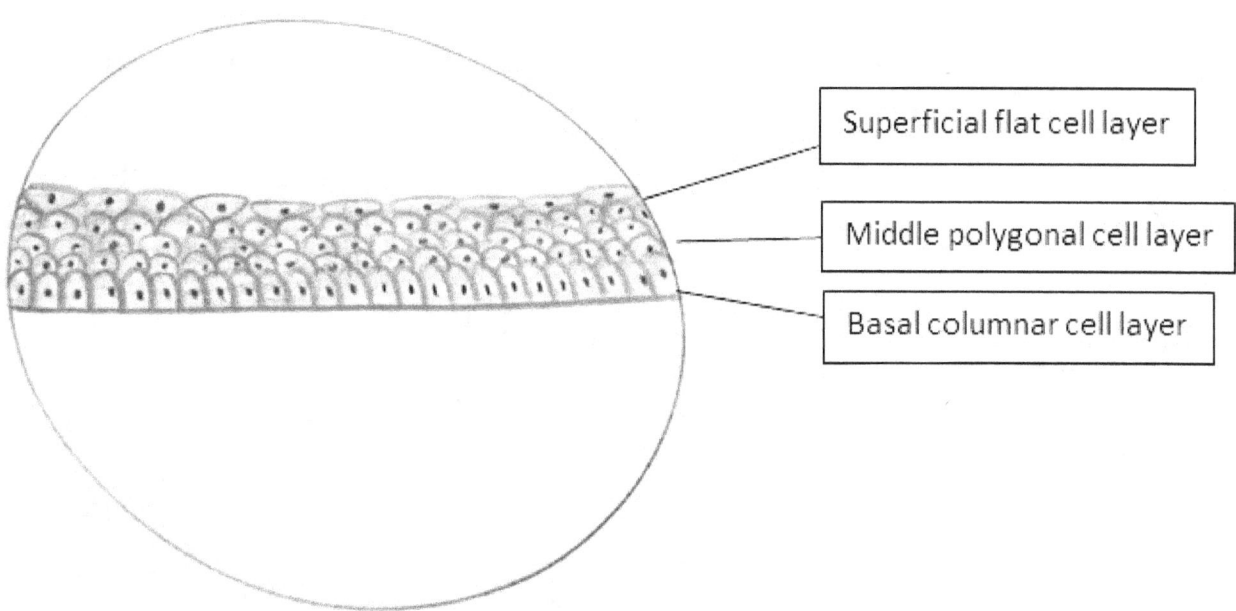

Superficial flat cell layer

Middle polygonal cell layer

Basal columnar cell layer

Stratified Squamous Non-Keratinized Epithelium: 8

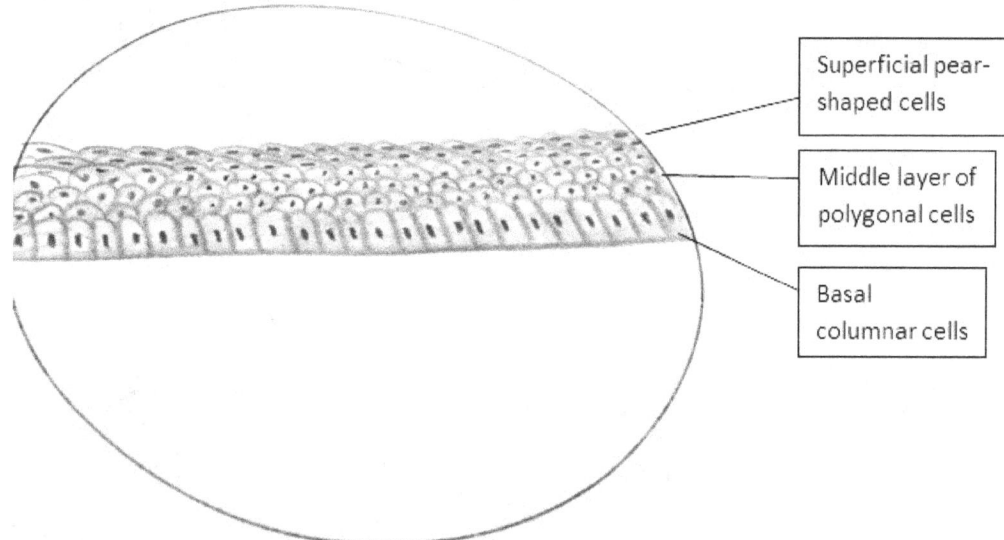

Superficial pear-shaped cells

Middle layer of polygonal cells

Basal columnar cells

Transitional Epithelium: 9

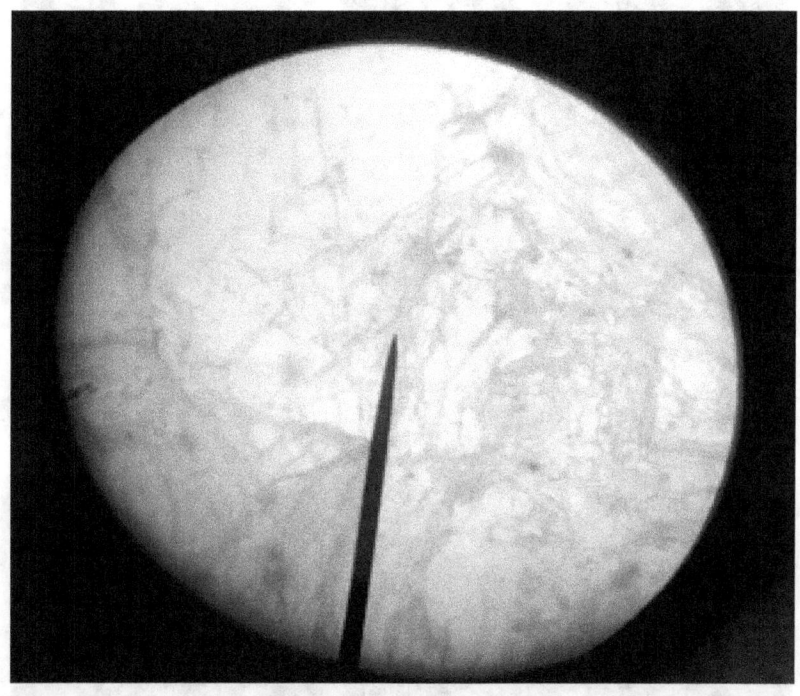

Loose Areolar Tissue: 1

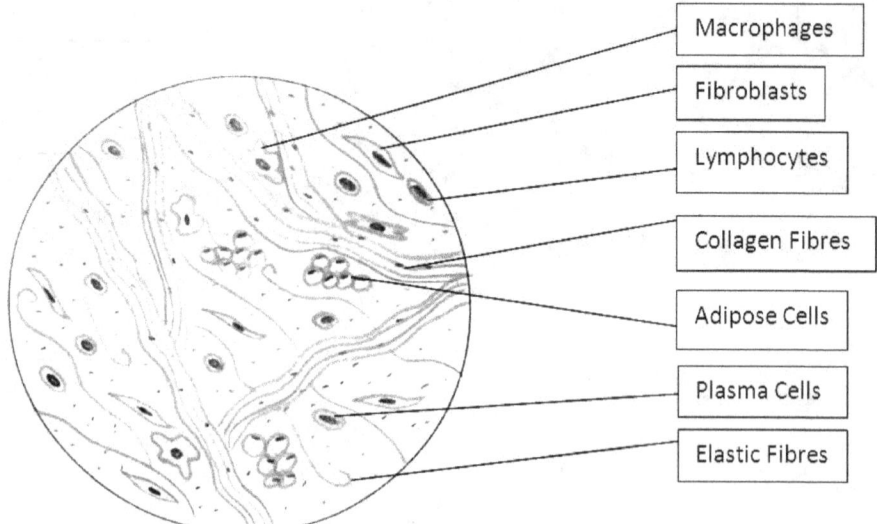

Macrophages

Fibroblasts

Lymphocytes

Collagen Fibres

Adipose Cells

Plasma Cells

Elastic Fibres

Loose Areolar Tissue: 2

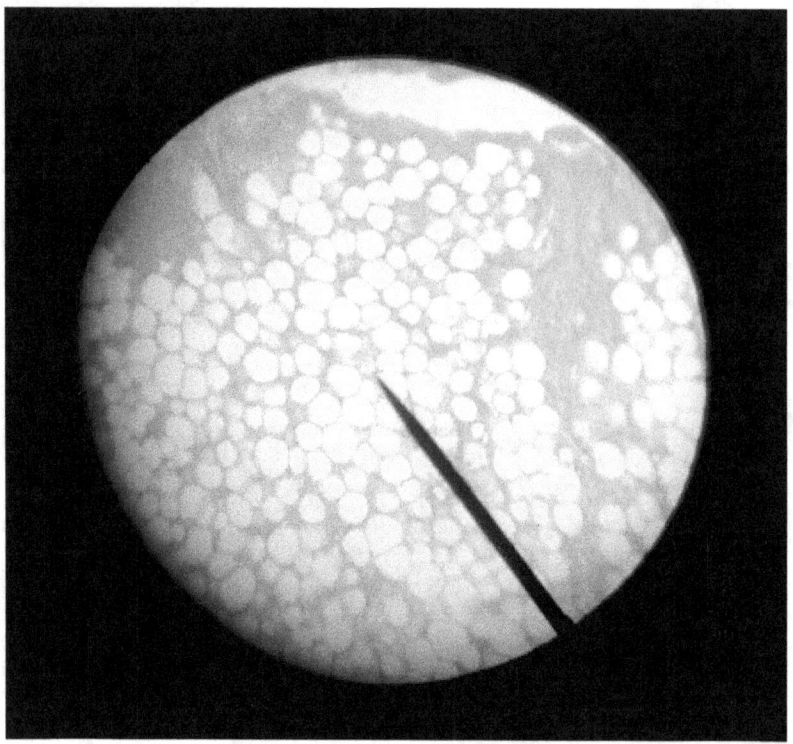

Adipose Tissue: 4

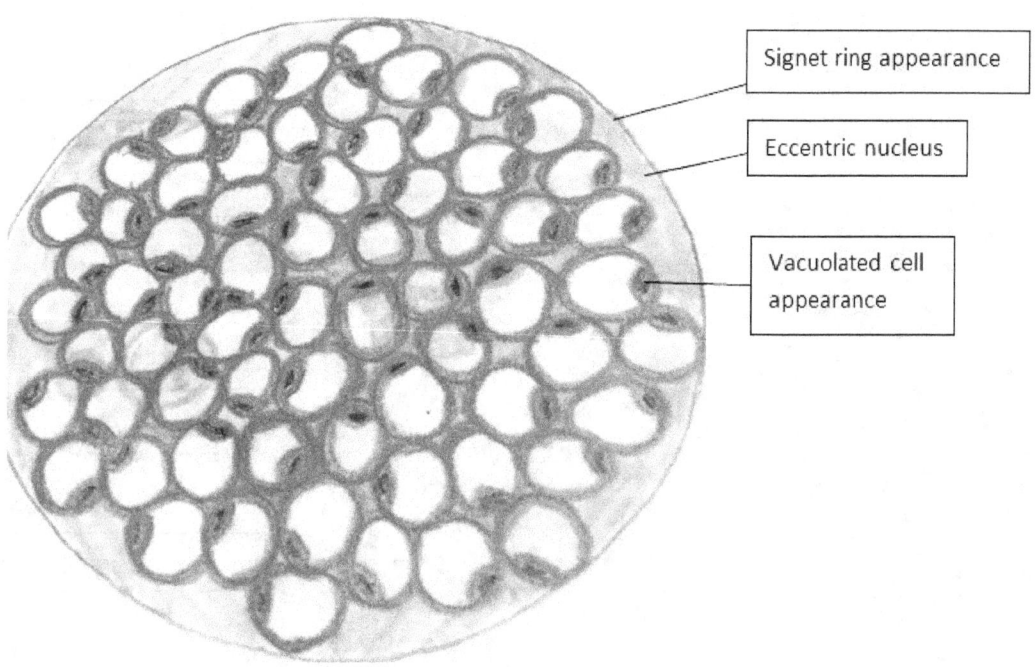

Signet ring appearance

Eccentric nucleus

Vacuolated cell appearance

Adipose Tissue: 5

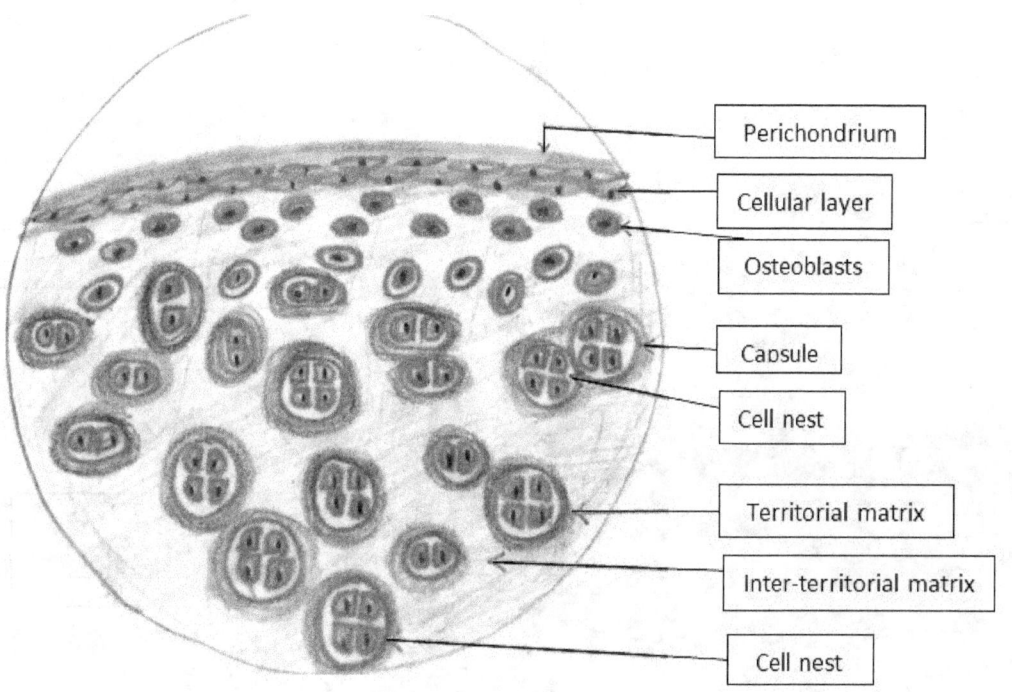

Perichondrium

Cellular layer

Osteoblasts

Capsule

Cell nest

Territorial matrix

Inter-territorial matrix

Cell nest

Hyaline Cartilage: 1

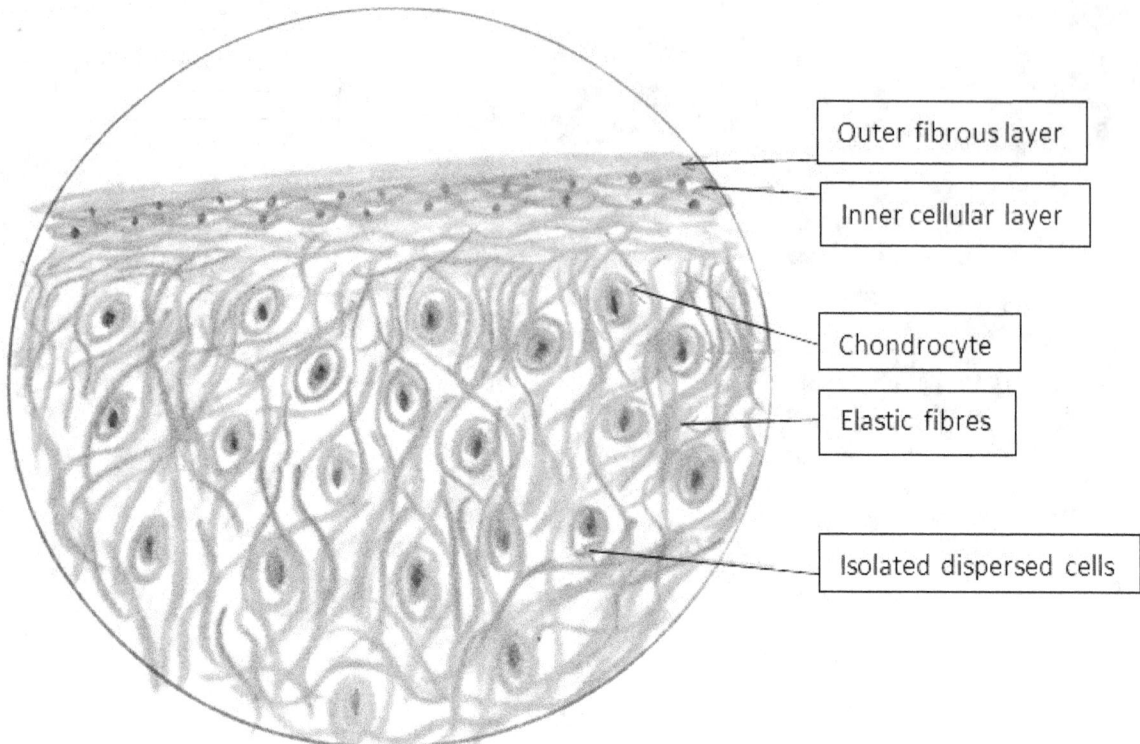

Outer fibrous layer

Inner cellular layer

Chondrocyte

Elastic fibres

Isolated dispersed cells

Elastic Cartilage: 2

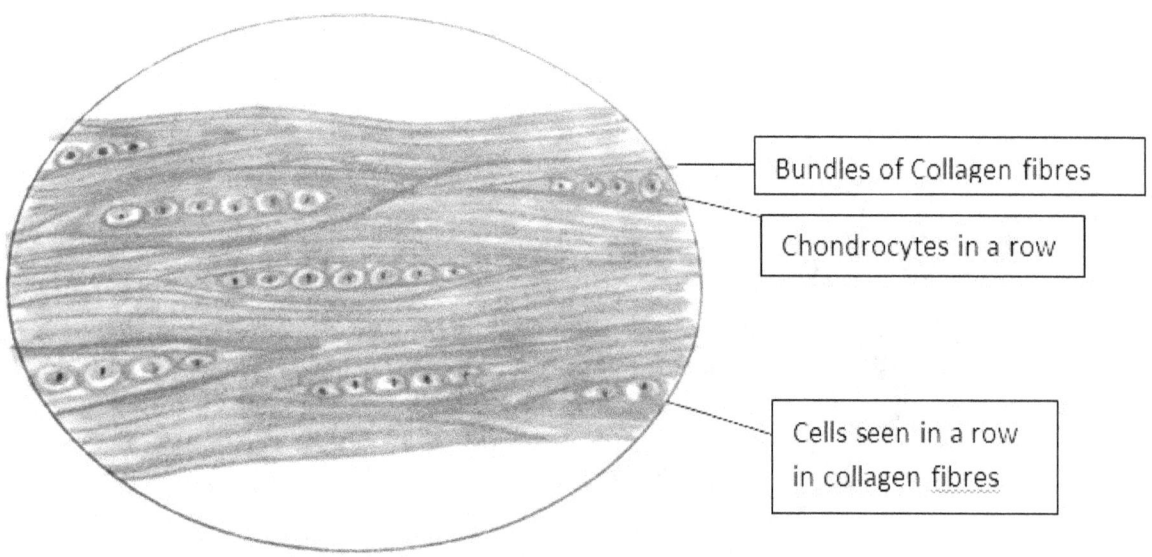

Bundles of Collagen fibres

Chondrocytes in a row

Cells seen in a row
in collagen fibres

White Fibro Cartilage: 3

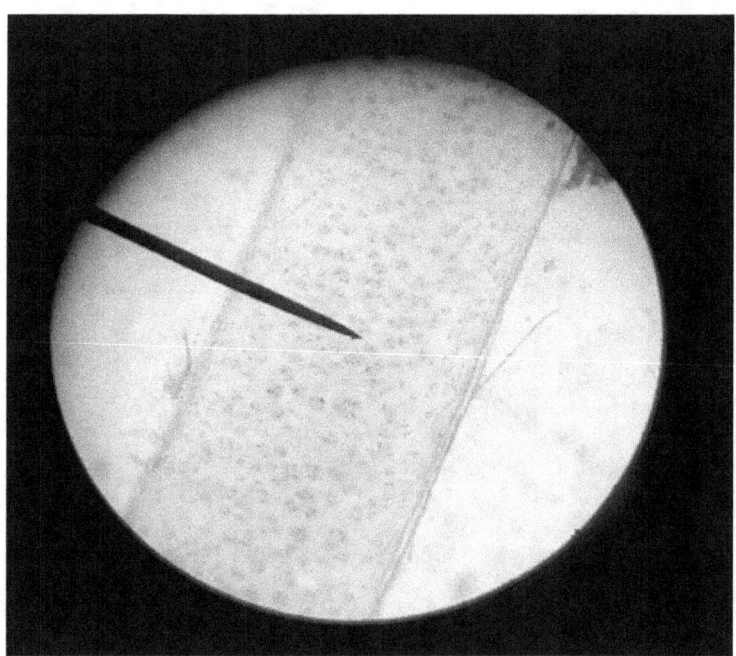

Hyaline Cartilage: 4

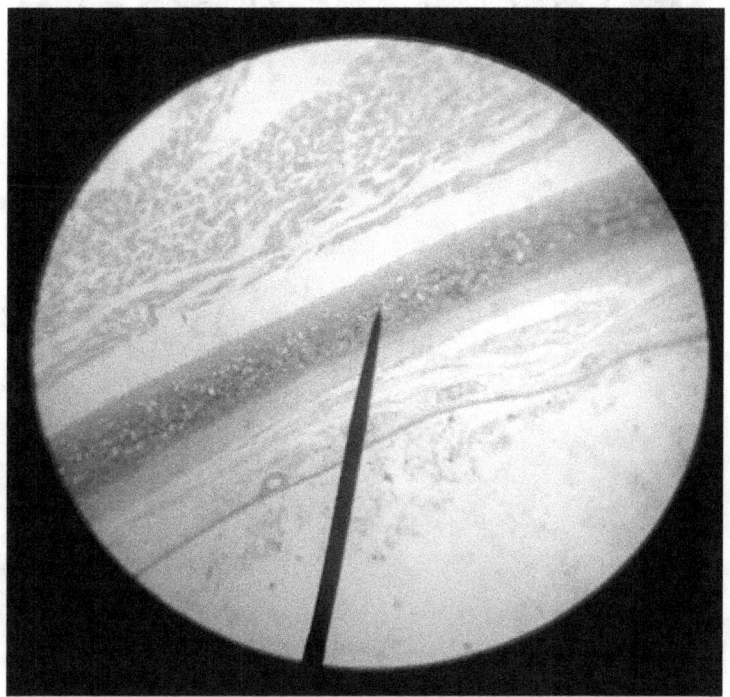

Elastic Cartilage: 6

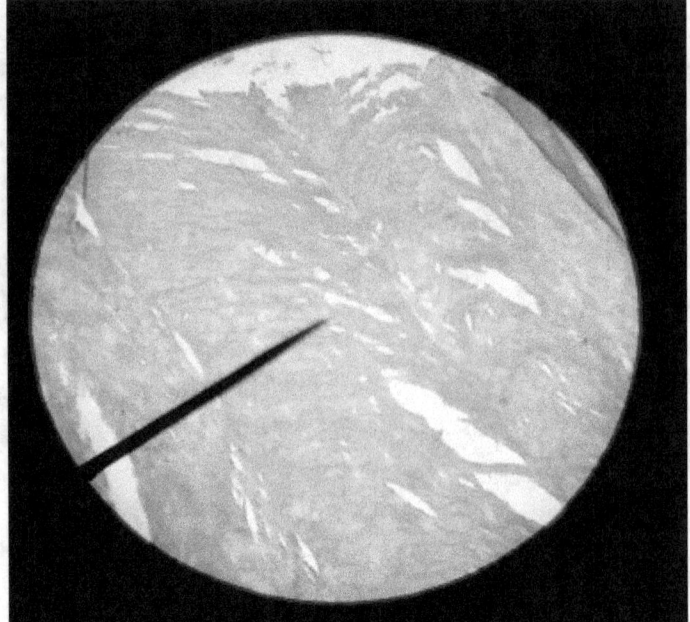

White Fibro – Cartilage: 8

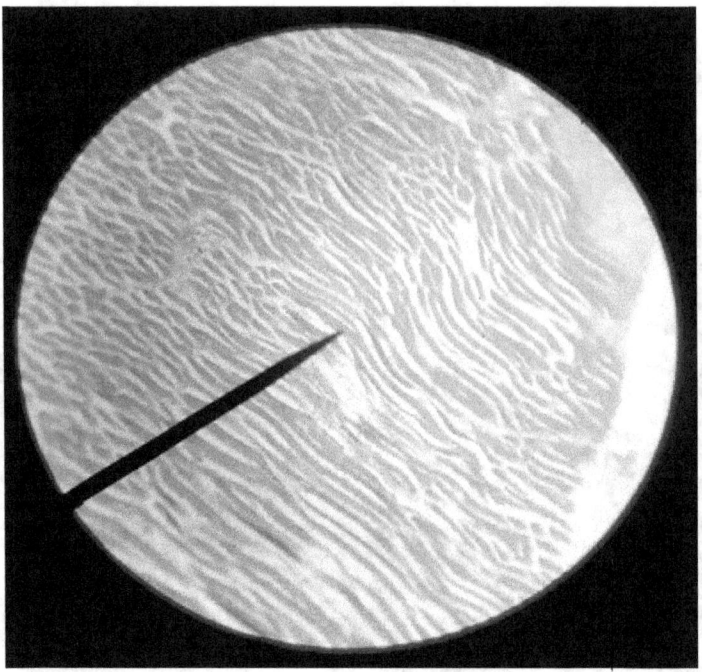

Skeletal Muscle: 3

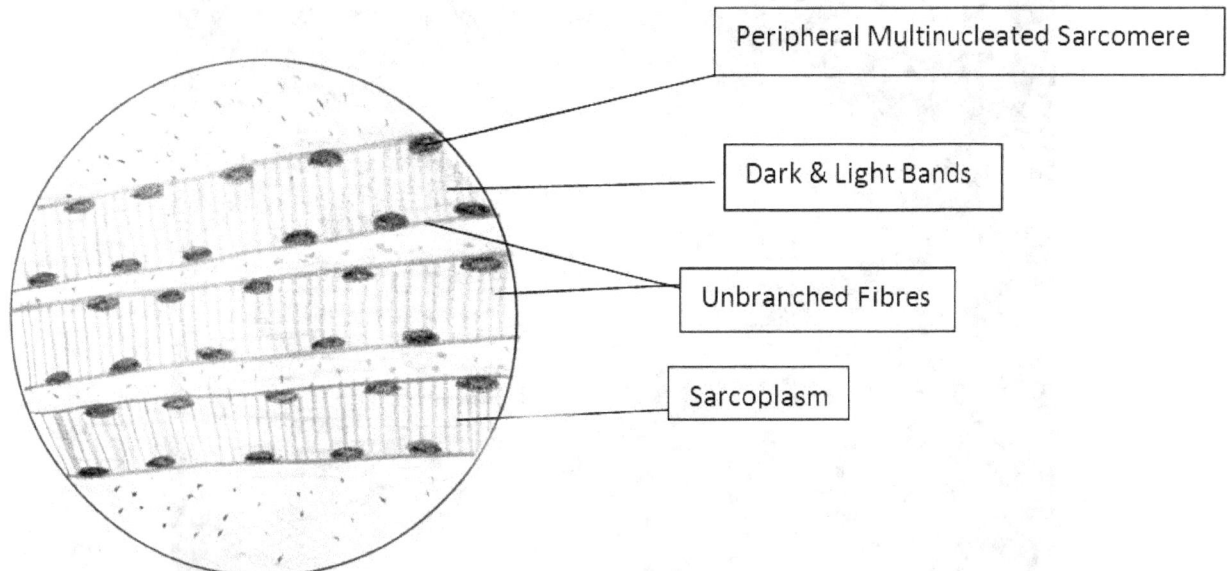

Peripheral Multinucleated Sarcomere

Dark & Light Bands

Unbranched Fibres

Sarcoplasm

Skeletal Muscle: 4

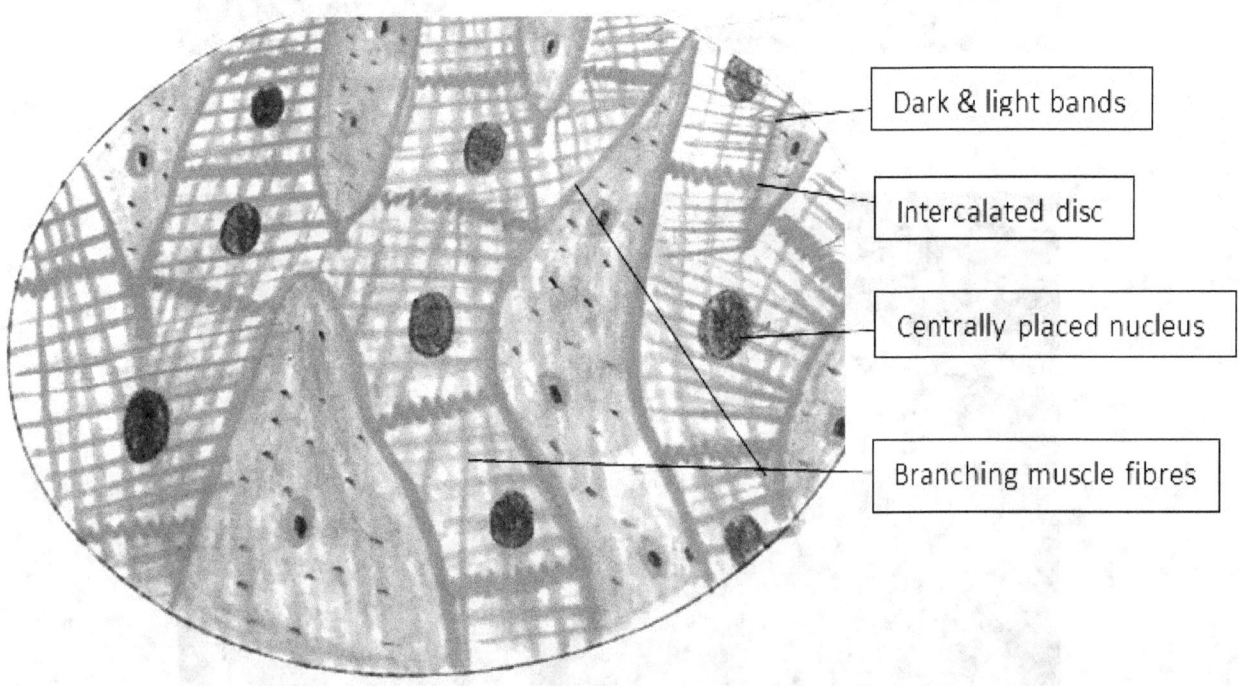

Dark & light bands

Intercalated disc

Centrally placed nucleus

Branching muscle fibres

Cardiac Muscle: 5

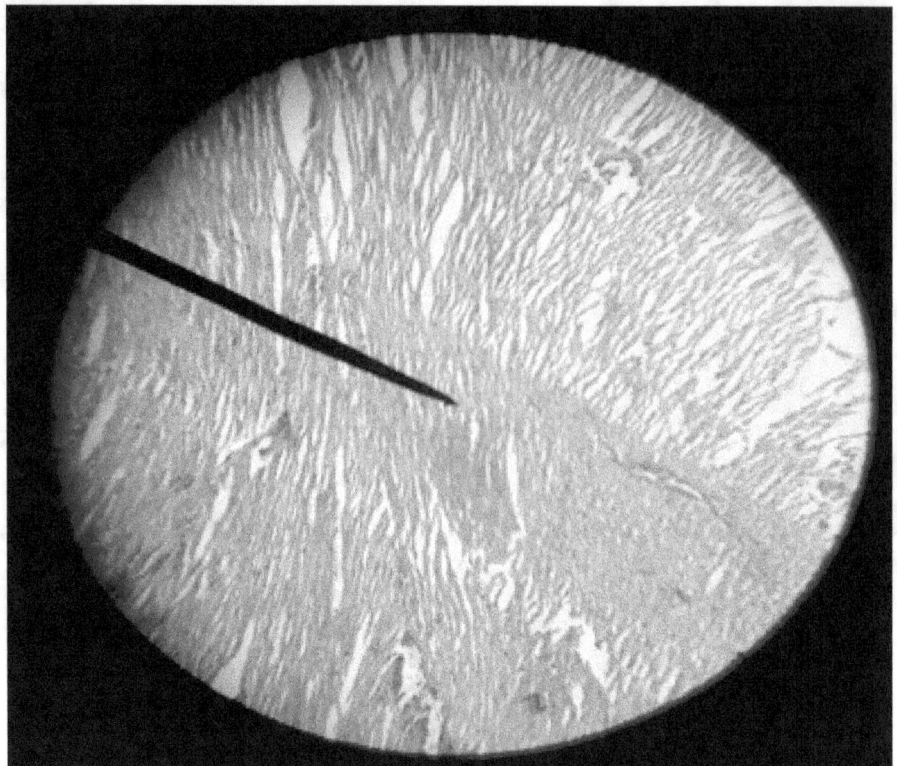

Cardiac Muscle: 6

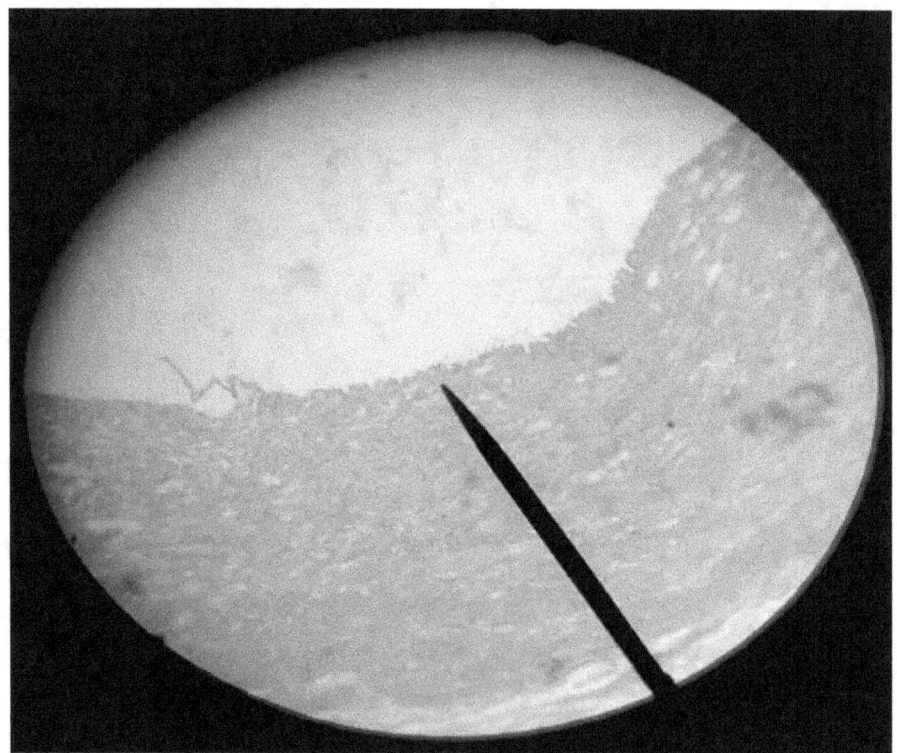

Large Sized Artery: 3

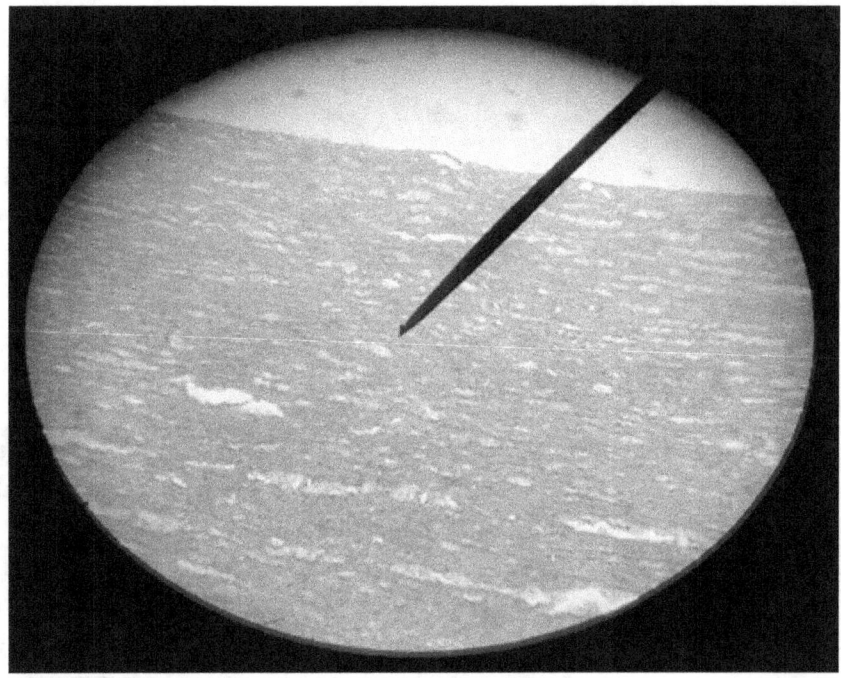

Medium Sized Artery: 4

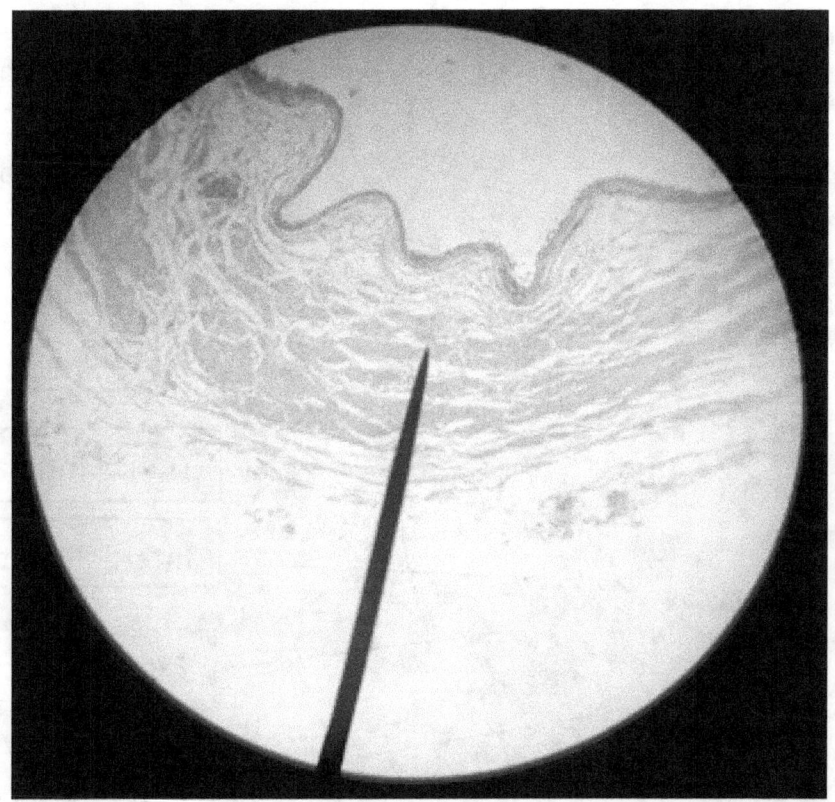

Large Sized Vein: 5

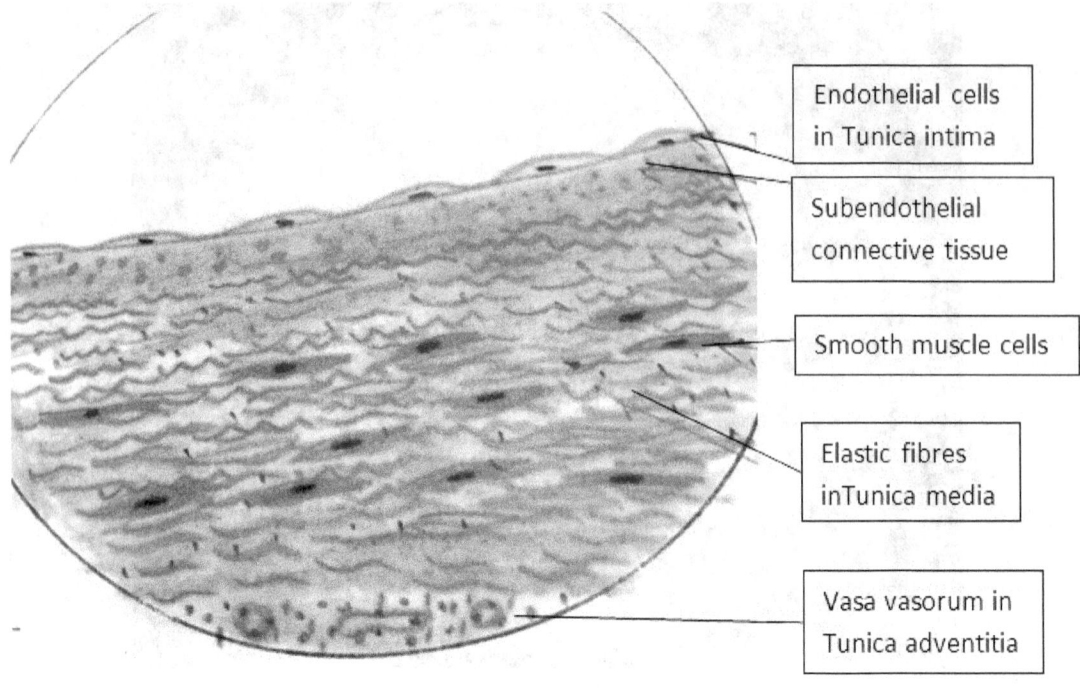

Large Sized Artery: 6

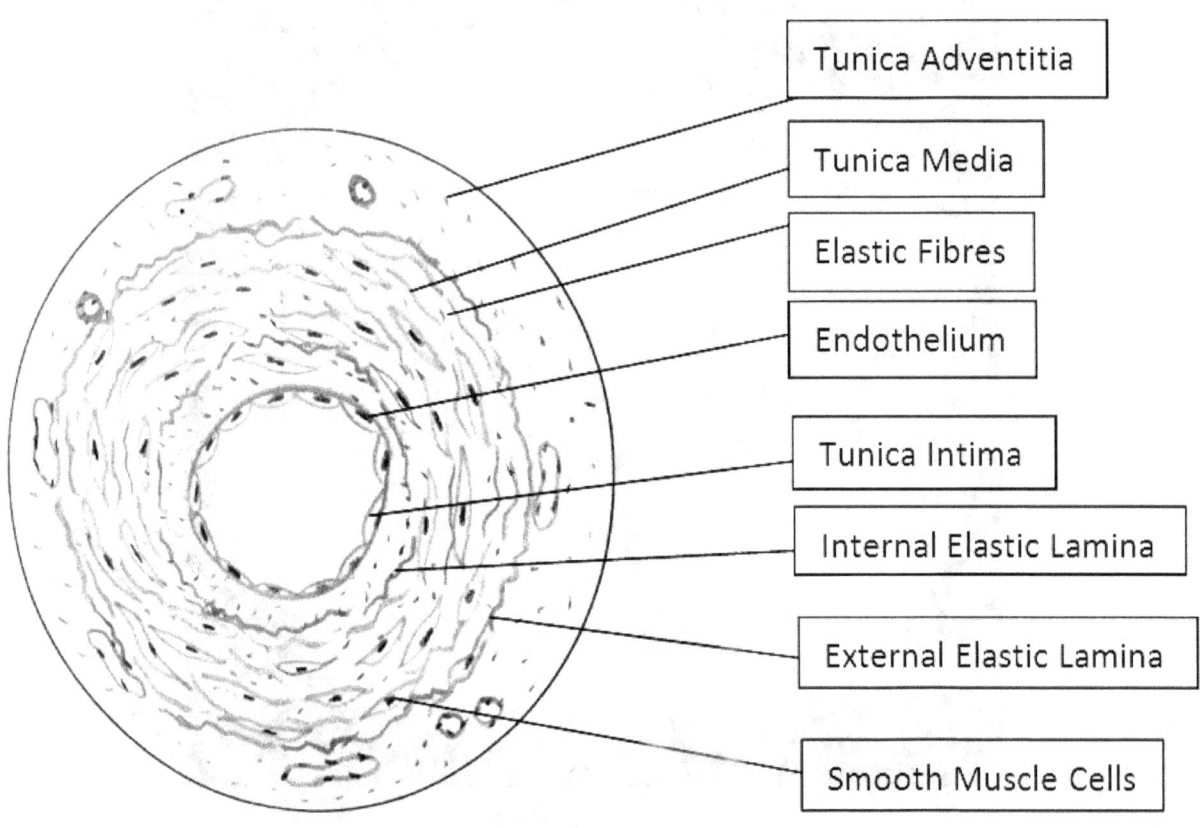

Medium Sized Artery: 7

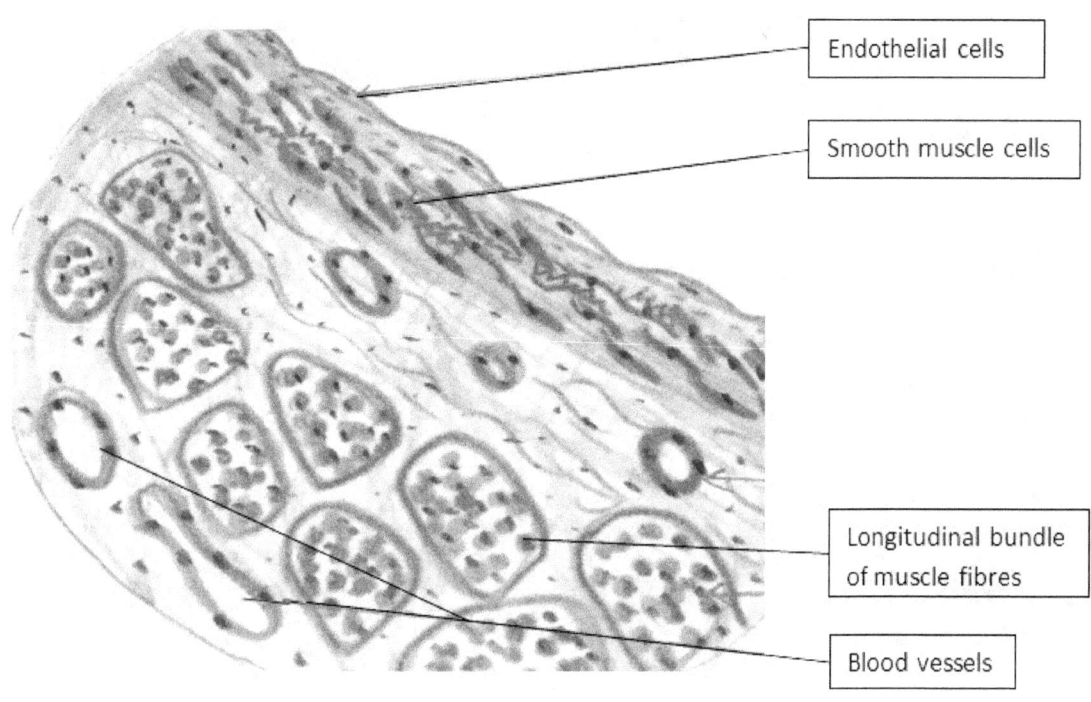

Endothelial cells

Smooth muscle cells

Longitudinal bundle of muscle fibres

Blood vessels

Large Sized Vein: 8

Chapter 12

LYMPHATIC SYSTEM

Objectives

1. Lymphstic system is very essential part of immune system in our body. Therefore, its basic structure and functions is very important to know.

2. Microcopic pictures of Lymph node, Palatine tonsil, Spleen and Thymus is frequently asked as short notes.

The **lymphatic system** consists of the **lymph capillaries, lymphatic vessels and lymph nodes**, it drains and filters the lymph. The lymph capillaries contain filtrate of blood plasma called as *tissue fluid,* which contains proteins, fat and bacteria. The lymph capillaries drain into lymph vessels which enter the lymph nodes, which act as filter for lymph and remove bacteria by phagocytosis, the lymphocytes produced by the lymph nodes are added to the lymph. The lymph nodes are bean-shaped structures found in various parts of the body like axillary LN, cervical LN, inguinal LN.

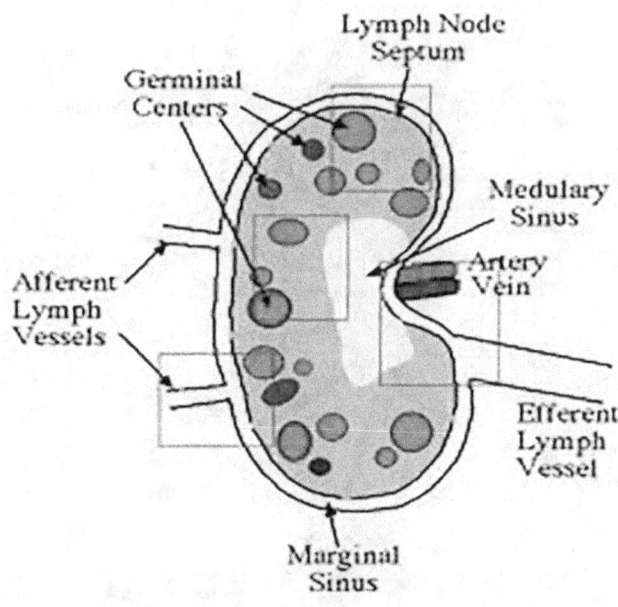

Lymphatic Vessels: 1

The Lymphatic System

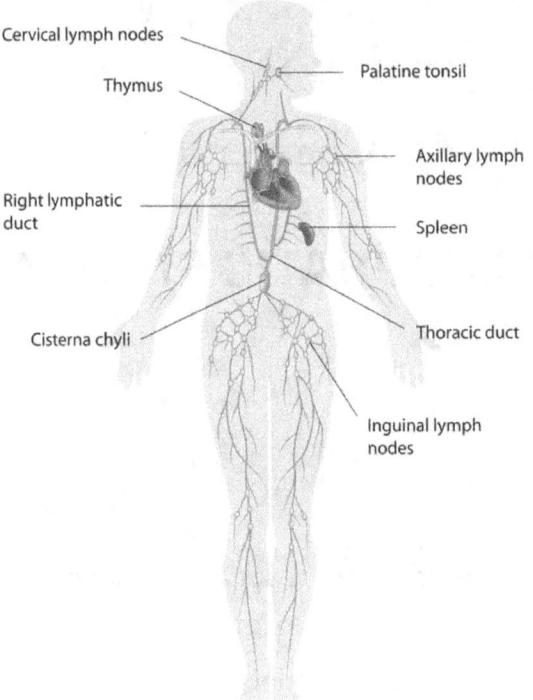

Lymphatic System: 2

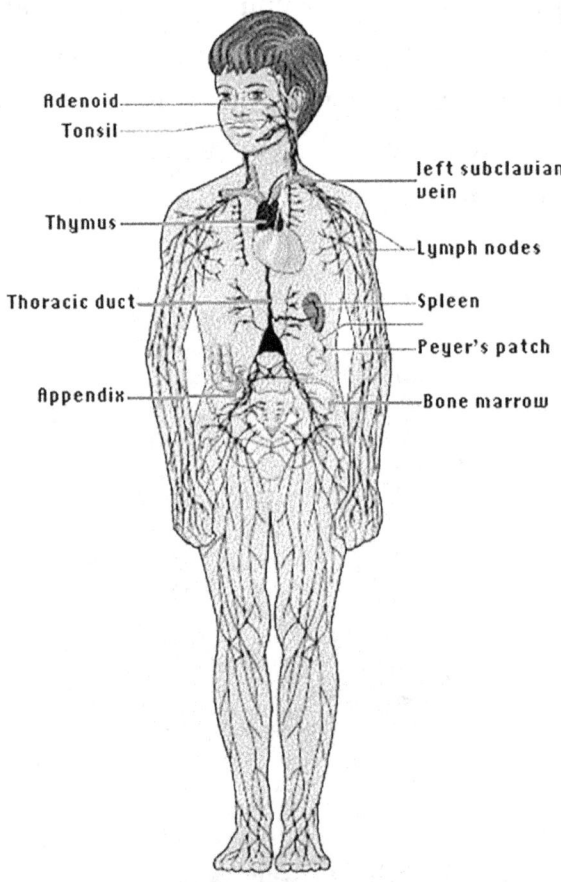

Lymphatic System: 3

Functions of Lymphatic System

*   Lymphatics drain large macro molecules like fat molecules, proteins, bacteria which cannot be drained by the blood capillaries.
*   Lymph nodes filter the bacteria by phagocytosis.
*   Lymph nodes are sites of production of lymphocytes.
*   Plasma cells of the lymph nodes produce antibodies in response to infection.

Lymphatics form a commonest route for the cancer cells to spread from one part to another. The LN become enlarged and painful, this is called as lymphadenitis/lympadenopathy.

Histology of Lymph Node

The lymph node has an outer darkly stained cortex and an inner lightly stained medulla. The cortex consists of lymphatic nodules made up of T and B lymphocytes, each nodule has a lightly stained area in the centre called as germinal centre, it has very few lymphocytes. The LN has a capsule, its connective tissue dips into the gland to form connective tissue septa/trabeculae, which divide the node into lobules. The hilum has blood vessels leaving/entering the LN.

The medulla consists of **medullary cords**, which are lymphocytes arranged in rows/columns. It contains **medullary sinuses** which are large capillaries. The medulla is highly vascular.

The sinuses are lined by endothelial cells and surrounded by pericytes and smooth muscle cells.

B lymphocytes help to destroy bacteria/foreign bodies (antigens) by producing antibodies/ immunoglobulins, this is called as **humoral immunity**, they also produce plasma cells. *T lymphocytes* help to identify specific antigens (virus, cancer cells), thus help in **cell mediated immunity.**

Apart from lymphocytes there are lymphoblasts, reticular cells, plasma cells, macrophages and blood vessels.

Applied Aspects

1. Inflammation and infection of Lymph nodes is called as Lymphadenitis, which can be localized or generalised. Enlarged lymphnodes are called as Lymphadenopathy, seen in metastasis of Breast Cancer, Tuberculosis, Syphilis and AIDS.
2. Inflammation of lymphatic vessels is called as Lymphangitis.
3. Lymphedema is swelling of particular regions due to lymphatic obstruction, as seen in Elephantiasis due Filarial parasite.

Histology of Lymph Node: 4 (for figure refer page no. 118)

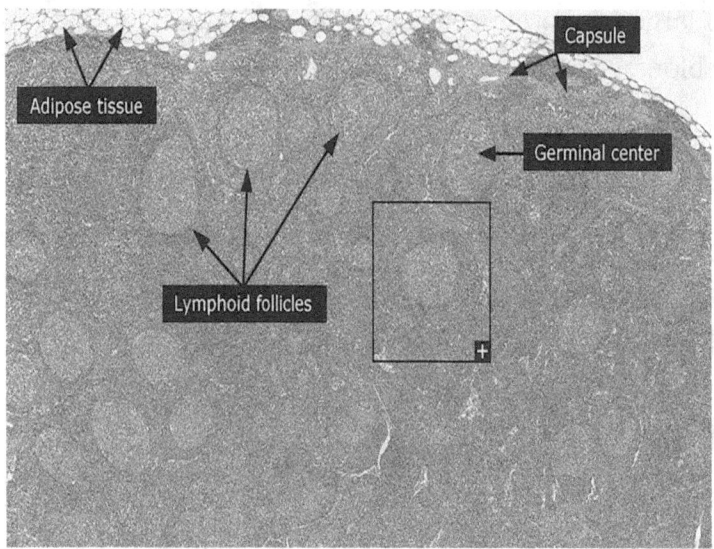

Lymph Node: 5

Lymph Node: 6 (for figure refer page no. 118)

Histology of Palatine Tonsil

The tonsil is lined by stratified squamous non-keratinized epithelium, which dips into the gland to form the tosillar crypts. It is made up of diffuse lymphatic tissue consisting of lymphatic nodules.

The tonsils become enlarged during infection called as *tonsillitis,* surgical removal of tonsils is called as *tonsillectomy.*

Histology of Palatine Tonsil: 7 (for figure refer page no. 119)

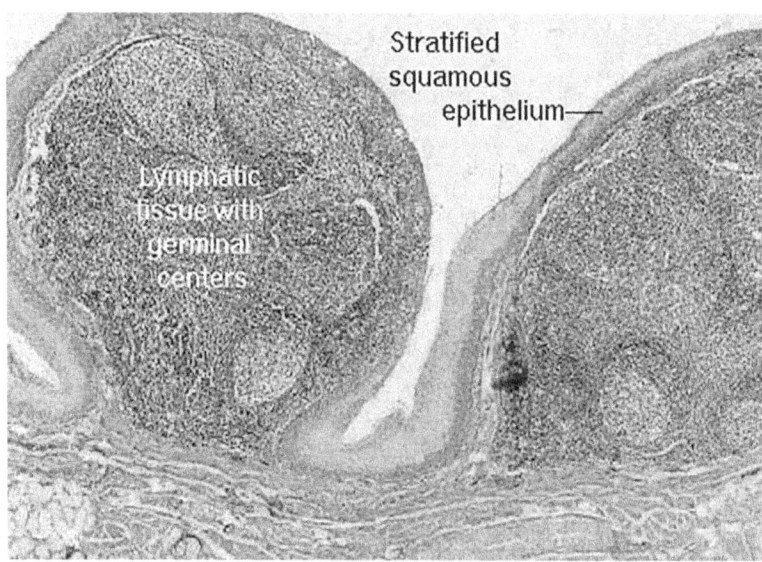

Histology of Palatine Tonsil: 8

Histology of Palatine Tonsil: 9 (for figure refer page no. 119)

Histology of Spleen

Spleen is the largest lymphoid organ in the body. It has a hilum for the blood vessels. Spleen is covered by capsule, the connective tissue septa/trabeculae extend into the gland to divide it into various lobules.

CIRCULATION THROUGH THE SPLEEN: The **Splenic artery** divides into **trabecular branches** which run in the septae, they then divide into **arterioles** which are surrounded by dense sheath of lymphocytes, these form the *white pulp*. The arterioles divide into **penicilli**, which show thickening in the walls called as **ellipsoids** (fibroblasts and macrophages), these ellipsoids open into the **ampulla** which drain into the reticular tissue, this is called as *red pulp*. This is called as *"open circulation."* If the blood drains into *the* sinusoids then into the veins in the trabeculae, this is called as *"closed circulation."*

WHITE PULP OF SPLEEN: White pulp consists of arteriole surrounded by a sheath of lymphocytes. The lymphatic nodules are called as "Malpighian bodies." Each nodule has a germinal centre and an eccentrically placed arteriole in the germinal centre. White pulp has both T and B lymphocytes.

RED PULP OF SPLEEN: Sinusoids are numerous, trabecular spaces are lined by reticular cells, inbetween the spaces are lymphocytes, macrophages, blood cells, these cells are arranged in cords called as "splenic cords of Billroth."

Applied Anatomy

Enlarged spleen is called as **splenomegaly,** seen in malaria, typhoid, etc. Removal of spleen is called as **splenectomy.**

Functions of Spleen

- B and T lymphocytes are produced, which maintain immunity of the body.
- Macrophages destroy bacteria/foreign particles by phagocytosis.
- In fetal life it's the site of production of all types of cells.
- Spleen stores blood when required.

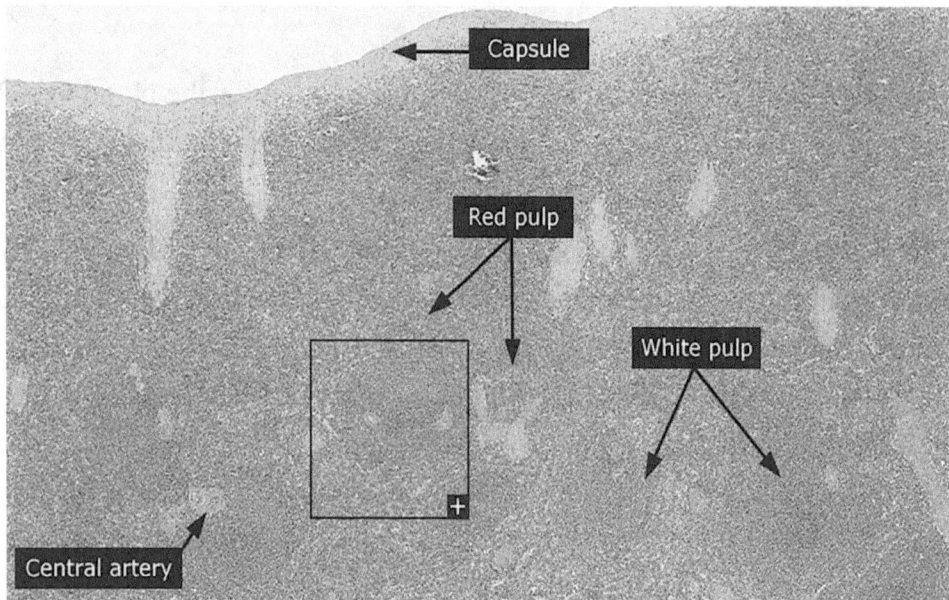

Histology of Spleen: 10

Histology of Spleen: 11 (for figure refer page no. 120)

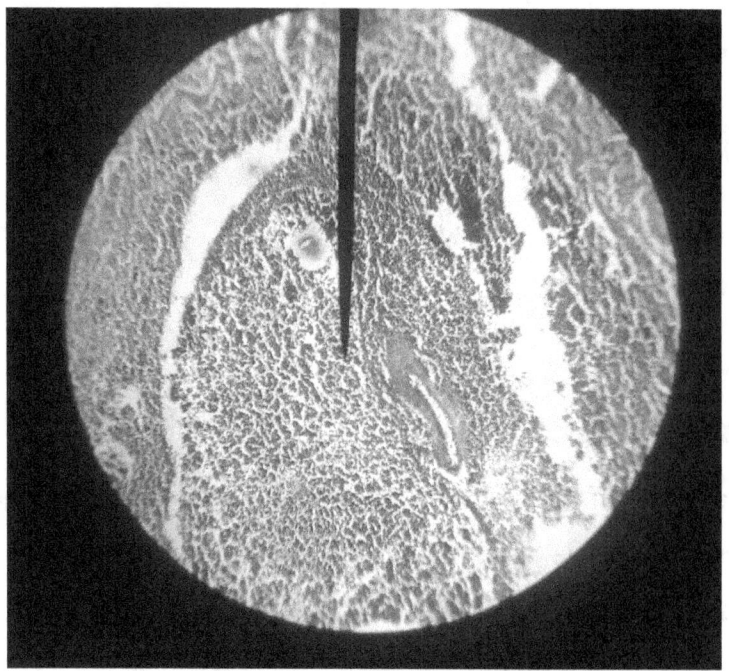

Histology of Spleen: 12

Histology of Spleen: 13 (for figure refer page no. 120)

Histology of Thymus

Thymus is a primary lymphoid organ seen in front of the neck, degenerates as age advances and converted into fat. Therefore, it is not seen in old age. It's the site of production of T lymphocytes.

Thymus consists of lymphatic tissue, it's capsule dips into the tissue to divide it into lobules, each lobule has its own cortex and medulla.

Types of cells seen in Thymus

1. *Epithelialcells/epitheliocytes;*

2. *Lymphocytes of thymus/thymocytes;*

3. *Macrophages and*

4. *Corpuscles of Hassall.*

   1. **Epitheliocytes:** Derived from endoderm, the cells are arranged in sheets, these sheets of cells form the blood-thymus barrier, their processes join other cells to form the reticulum. Epitheliocytes promote T-cell differentiation and proliferation. Types of epitheliocytes are:

      Type-1: Present around the blood vessels, septa and capsule;

      Type-2 & 3: Present in the outer and inner cortex.

      Type-4: Seen in the deep part of the cortex and medulla.

      Type-5: Seen around the Hassall's corpuscles.

   2. **Thymocytes/Lymphocytes:** The cortex is densely filled with lymphocytes, where as the medulla has few lymphocytes.

   3. **Macrophages:** These are seen below the capsule and in the medulla, they help in phagocytosis.

   4. **Hassall's Corpuscles:** Present in the medulla, they are small, having a central core of degenerated epithelial cells with macrophages, which appear as pink staining hyaline mass, around this mass is the concentrically arranged epithelial cells (onion ring appearance).

Functions of Thymus

♦ Thymus is a primary lymphoid organ for the production of T lymphocytes, it's the site where the lymphocytes multiply and mature into immunocompetent T lymphocytes, these then migrate to secondary lymphoid organs like lymphnodes, spleen and tonsils.

♦ Thymus produces hormones like thymulin, thymopoietin, thymosin alpha 1 and thymosin beta 4, these hormones help in stimulating and controlling the multiplication of the lymphocytes.

Applied Anatomy: Thymus is enlarged in *Myasthenia gravis,* wherein, the skeletal muscles become weak, here the immune system attacks it's own body proteins (autoimmune disease), removal of thymus improves the condition.

Histology of Thymus: 14 (for figure refer page no. 121)

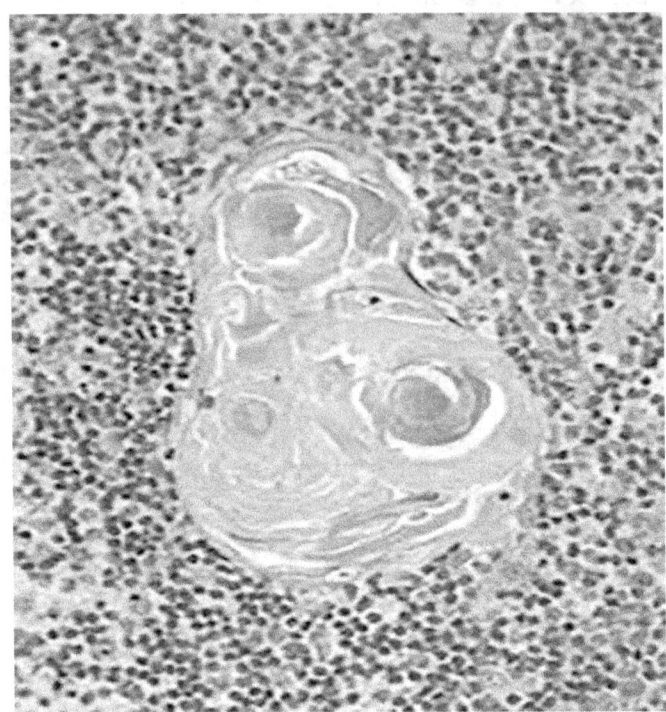

Histology of Thymus: 15 (Hassall's Corpuscles)

Histology of Thymus: 16 (for figure refer page no. 121)

Multiple Choice Questions

1. All of the following are the Secondary lymphoid organs except:

   a. Tonsil;

   b. Spleen;

   c. Thymus;

   d. Lymphnode.

   (Answer: c)

2. Hassall's corpuscles are characteristic of:

   a. Lymphnode;

   b. Thymus;

   c. Spleen;

   d. Tonsil.

   (Answer: b)

3. Lymphadenopathy is seen in:

   a. Malignancy;

   b. Tuberculosis;

   c. AIDS;

   d. All of the above.

   (Answer: d)

Model Questions

Short Notes (5 Marks)

1. Describe the microscopic picture of Thymus.

2. Enumerate the functions of Lymphnode and draw a neat labeled diagram of histology of lymphnode.

3. Microscopic picture of Palatine Tonsil.

4. Histology of Spleen.

Chapter 13

NERVOUS SYSTEM

Objectives

1. The classification of Neurons is important, the structure and functions of Nervous tissue must be known in order to understand the Physiology of Nerve impulses.

2. To know the difference between the microscopic appearance of Optic nerve and Peripheral nerve is important.

Definition: The Nervous tissue is a specialized tissue for conduction of impulses, the structural and functional unit of nervous tissue is the **Neuron**, and its connective tissue is called as the **Neuroglia**.

Structure of Neuron: Neuron has a cell body and cell processes called as axon and dendrites. Nucleus is large and spherical. Cytoplasm shows Nissl's body, which consists of ER and ribosomes. The axon is covered with myelin sheath for conduction of impulses, its dilated upper end is called as axon hillock.

Each nerve fibre is covered with neurilemma or sheath of Schwann, the myelin sheath is laid by the Schwann cells in the peripheral nervous tissue and by oligodendrocytes in CNS. The myelin sheath shows intervals called as Node of Ranvier, the impulses are conducted from one node to another. The myelin sheath increases the velocity of impulse conduction.

The nervous connective tissue called as Neuroglia which consists of cells like astrocytes, microglia, oligodendrocytes, ependymal cells, satellite cells and Schwann cells.

Structure of a Typical Neuron

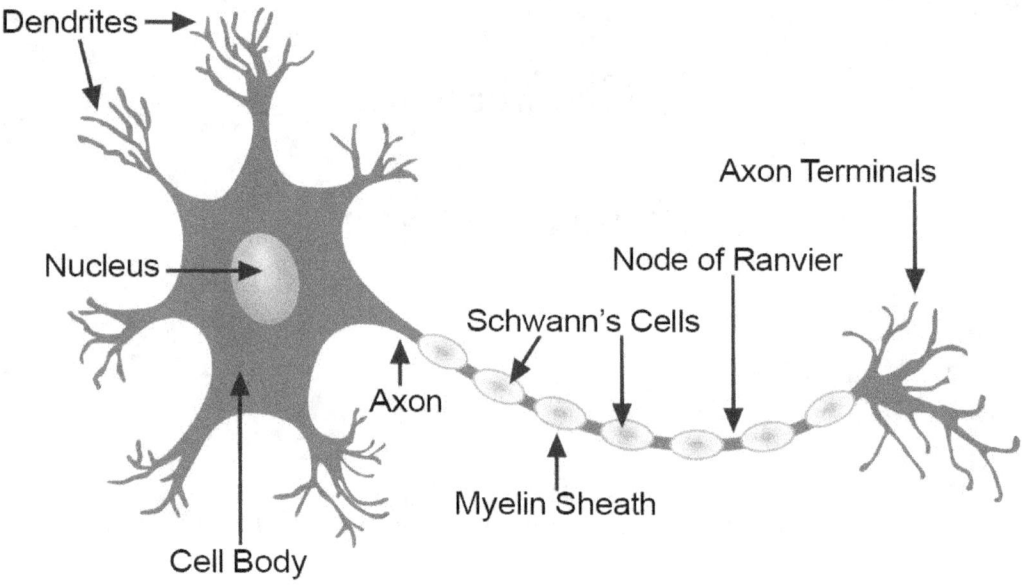

Structure of Neuron: 1

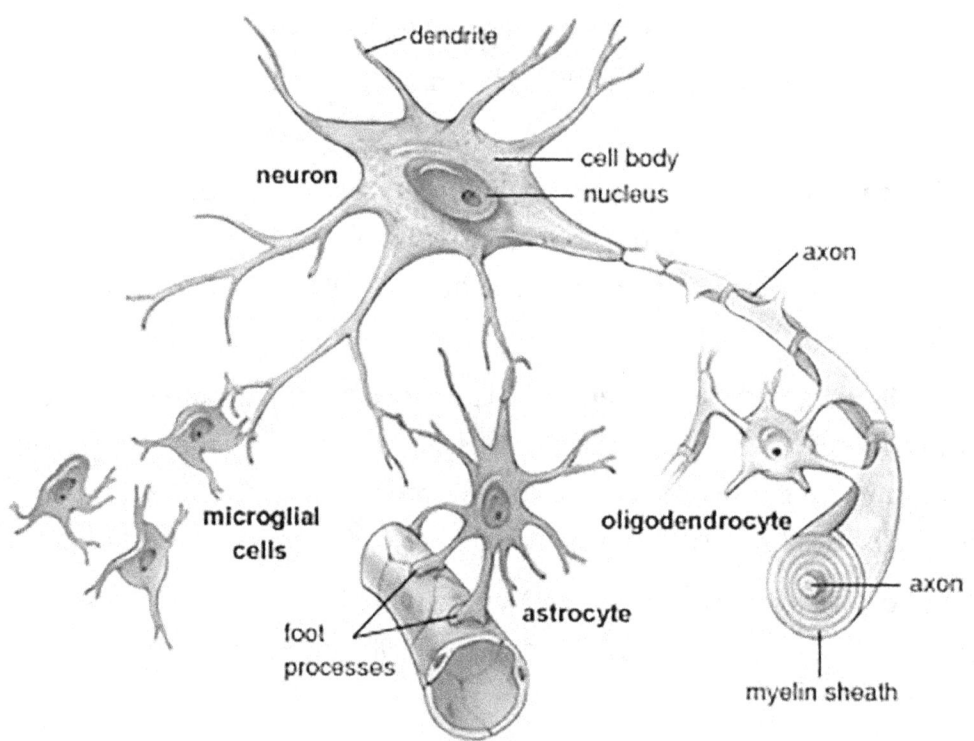

Cells of Nervous Tissue: 2

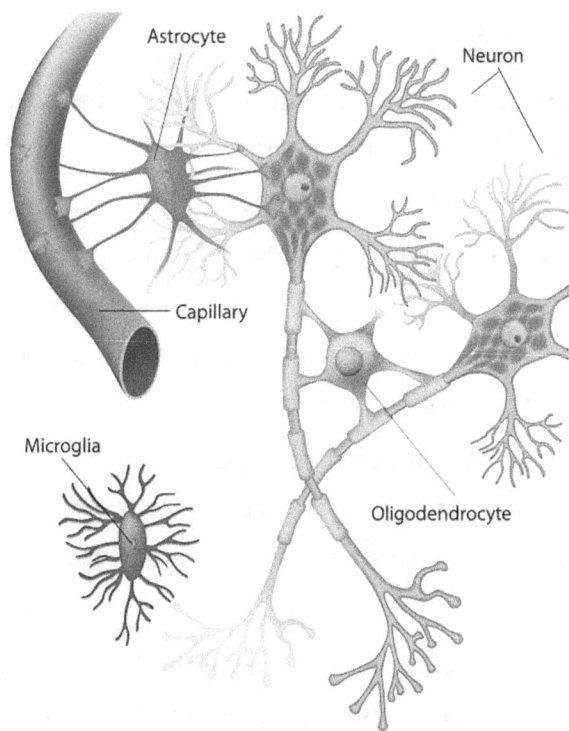

Cells of Nervous Tissue: 3

NERVOUS SYSTEMS: The brain and the spinal cord form the **CNS** whereas; the spinal cord forms the **PNS**. The peripheral nervous system consists of cranial and spinal nerves. It is divided into:

a. **Somatic N S:** Supplies the head, neck, trunk and limbs;

b. **Autonomic N S:** Supplies the viscera, blood vessels and glands.

c. **Enteric N S:** Supplies the gut/GIT.

Classification of Nervous Tissue

Depending on the number of processes:

1. **Unipolar Neurons:** Neuron has a single cell process e.g. trigeminal nucleus in mid brain.

2. **Bipolar Neurons:** Axons and dendrites arise from the opposite poles of the neuron e.g. olfactory cells.

3. **Multipolar Neurons:** Neuron show one axon and many dendrites e.g. sympathetic ganglion.

4. **Pseudounipolar Neurons:** A single process of neuron divides into two, an axon and a dendrite e.g. sensory and cranial ganglia.

Depending on Functions

1. **Sensory/Receptor Neurons:** e.g. bipolar neurons/pseudo-unipolar neurons, these lie outside the CNS, brain and spinal nerves act as sensory receptors for touch, pain and temperature.

2. **Inter-Neurons/Internuncial Neurons:** Sensory impulses are carried by these neurons from the brain to analyze and act accordingly; these connect the sensory to motor neurons, e.g. multipolar neurons.

3. **Motor Neurons:** These neurons carry the response of the impulse from the brain/spinal cord to the effector organ, e.g. multipolar neurons.

NERVES: A Nerve consists of large number of fibres/axons which is binded by the connective tissue. The nervous system consists of brain, cranial nerves (12 pairs, which supply the head and neck regions), spinal cord and spinal nerves (31 pairs, which supply the right and left sides of the body).

The nerve fibres carrying the nerve impulses from the brain/spinal cord to various parts of the body are called as the **efferent fibres/motor fibres.** The fibres carrying sensory impulses from skin to CNS are called as **afferent fibres/sensory fibres.**

HISTOLOGY OF PERIPHERAL NERVE: The peripheral nerve consists of bundle of nerve axons/fibres held together by connective tissue. Whereas, the collection of cell bodies present outside the CNS are called as the ganglia.

Each nerve fibre is covered by neurilemmal sheath called as *endoneurium*. The nerve bundles are covered by *perineurium*, whereas, the whole nerve trunk is covered by *epineurium*. The epineurium contains the blood vessels and lymphatics. The peripheral nerve consists of both motor and sensory neurons.

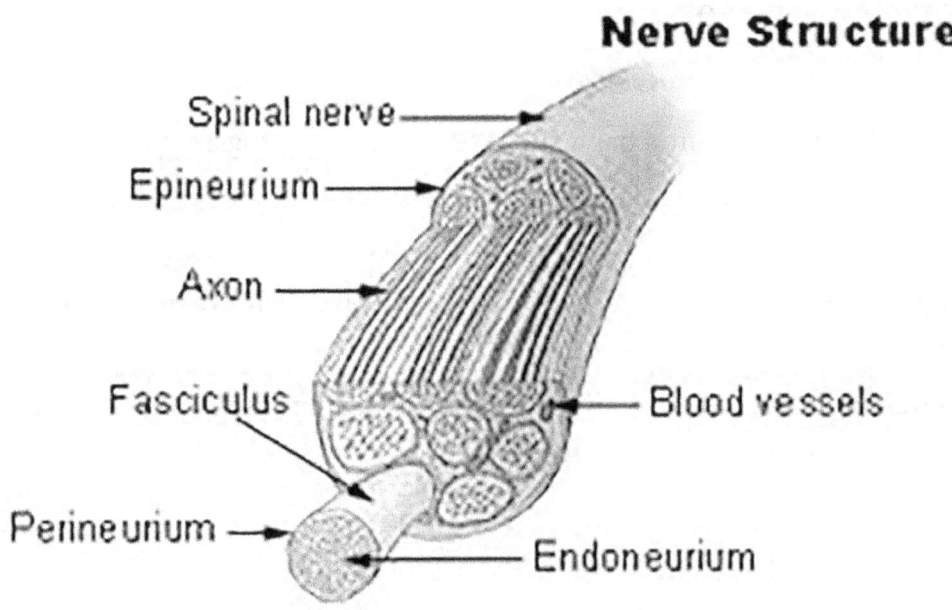

Coverings of Nerve Bundle: 4

Histology of Peripheral Nerve: 5 (for figure refer page no. 122)

Peripheral Nerve: 6 (for figure refer page no. 122)

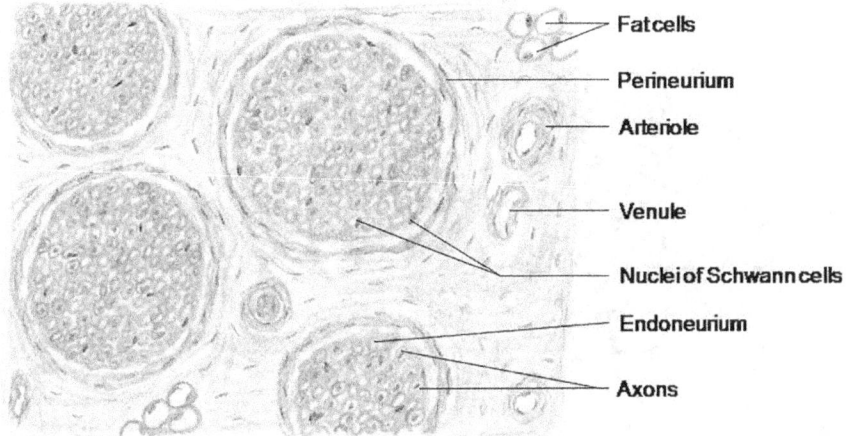

Fat cells
Perineurium
Arteriole
Venule
Nuclei of Schwann cells
Endoneurium
Axons

Peripheral Nerve: 7

Histology of Optic Nerve

The optic nerve (4 cms) is made up of axons of ganglion cells from retina, cross section of the nerve shows central retinal artery and vein in the centre of the nerve. Surrounding this are the c/s of axons which form a thick nerve bundle, this is divided into nerve fasciculi by the piamater. The nerve is covered by outer **dura mater,** middle **arachnoid mater** and the inner **pia mater.** The cell bodies of these neurons are present in the retina.

The optic nerve derives its coverings from the white matter of the brain, from the stalk of the optic vesicle. Myelination is derived from the oligodendroglia. It is devoid of endoneurium and if damaged cannot regenerate. The pial sheath carrying blood vessels projects into the nerve as numerous septa and divides it into 800–1000 bundles of polygonal areas.

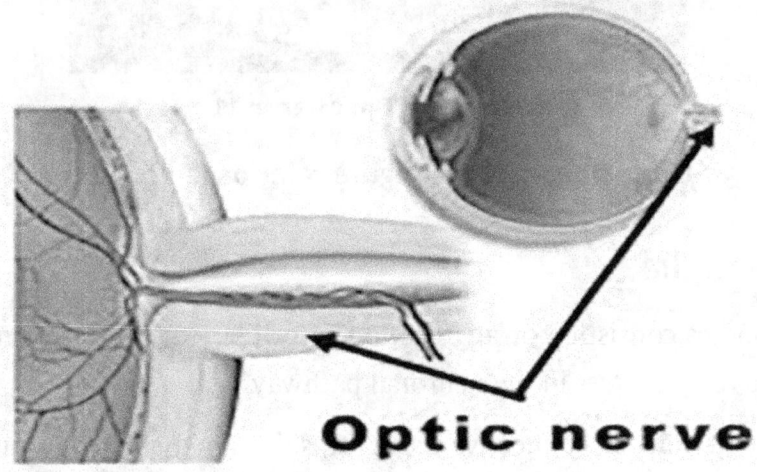

Optic nerve

Optic Nerve: 8

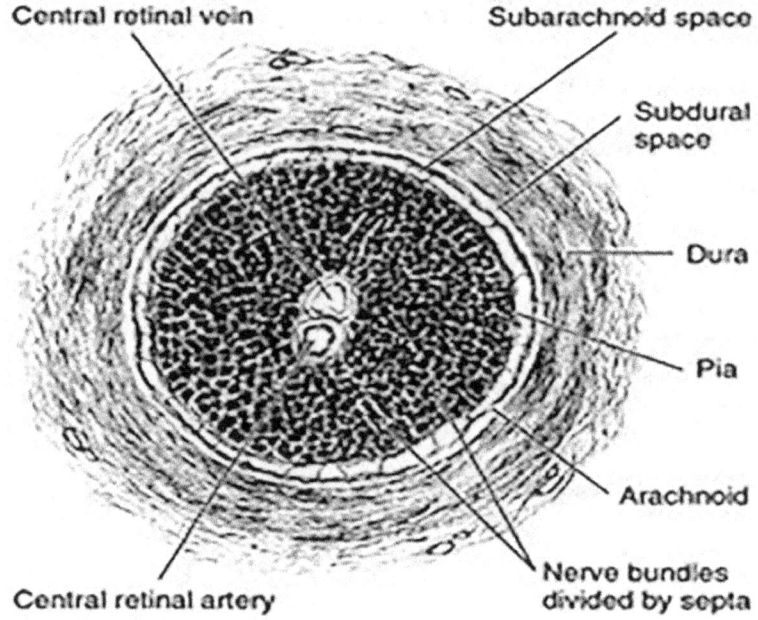

Central retinal vein
Subarachnoid space
Subdural space
Dura
Pia
Arachnoid
Nerve bundles divided by septa
Central retinal artery

Cross Section of Optic Nerve: 9

Histology of Optic Nerve: 10 (for figure refer page no. 123)

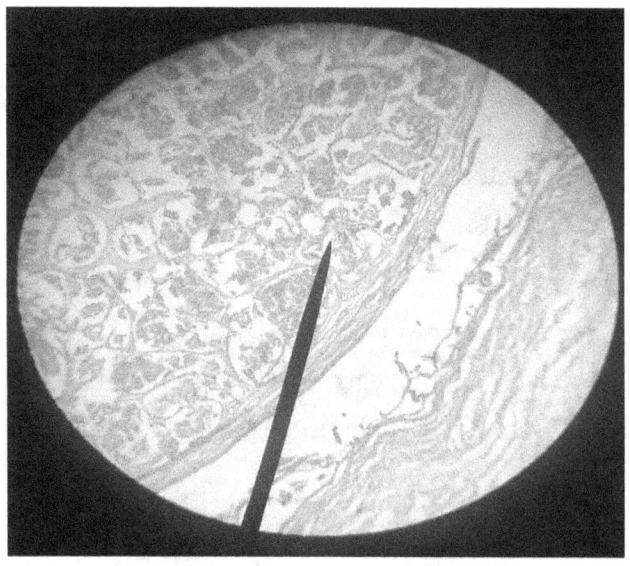

Coverings of Optic Nerve: 11

Optic Nerve: 12 (for figure refer page no. 123)

Histology of Ganglia

Ganglia are oval bodies consisting of aggregation of cell bodies/cytons of neurons outside the CNS. They serve as relay cantres in the neuronal pathway.

They are covered by dense connective tissue capsule called as epineurium. Each cell has a layer of flat cells around it called as **satellite cells**, these act as supporting cells and help in insulation, and are seen only in the PNS. They also provide pathway for metabolic exchange.

There are Two Types of Ganglia

1. Sensory/spinal/somatic/dorsal root ganglion;
2. Motor/autonomic ganglion (sympathetic/parasympathetic).

Sensory Ganglion

It is covered by capsule called as epineurium.

There are pseudo-unipolar neurons arranged in groups, they are separated by bundles of myelinated nerve fibres running in various directions.

The neurons are large, round of various sizes, with centrally placed nucleus in the perikaryon.

The cells are surrounded by well defined flat capsular supporting cells called as satellite cells.

Sensory Ganglion: 13 (for figure refer page no. 124)

Sensory Ganglion: 14 (for figure refer page no. 124)

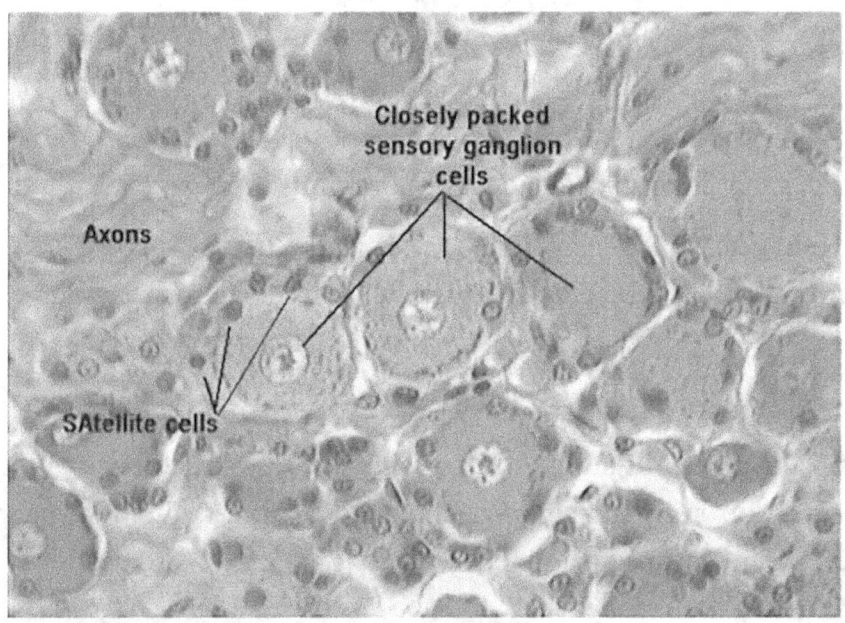

Sensory Ganglion: 15

Autonomic Ganglion

The ganglion is covered by capsule called as epineurium.

There are multipolar neurons which are small, angular and of uniform sizes with eccentrically placed nucleus.

The calls are scattered, isolated, widely spaced and diffuse.

The satellite cells are not well defined, less in number and irregularly placed.

The nerve fibres are non-myelinated and thinner, and are scattered in between the cells.

Autonomic Ganglion: 16 (for figure refer page no. 125)

Autonomic Ganglion: 17 (for figure refer page no. 125)

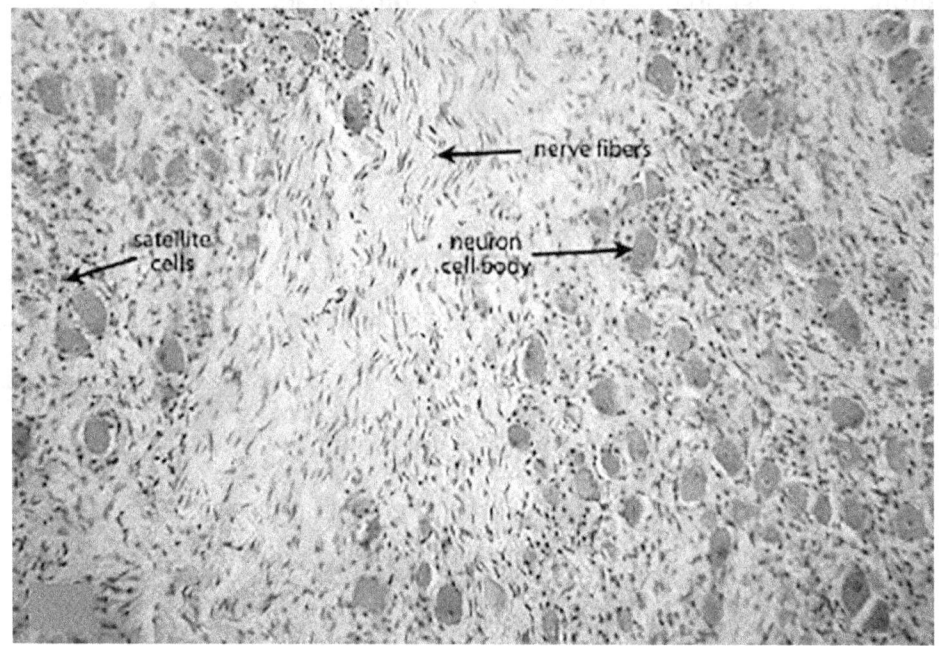

Autonomic Ganglion: 18

The autonomic ganglia are sympathetic and parasympathetic ganglia.

The sympathetic ganglia are seen along the sympathetic chain, along side of the vertebral column, the neuronal cytoplasm synthesizes catechol-amines(neurotransmitter). They are related the spinal segments like:

e.g. Superior and inferior cervical ganglion.

The **parasympathic ganglia** are related to the glandular structures like the otic ganglion, pterygopalatine ganglion, submandibular ganglion and ciliary ganglion, the neuronal cytoplasm synthesizes acetylcholine (neurotransmitter).

Applied Aspects

1. In cases of Leprosy the nerve fibres degenerate and damage to the Schwann cells is seen.

2. Any injury to the Peripheral nerves will lead to Paralysis of the muscles it supplies.

3. Complete damage to the Optic nerve will lead to total blindness.

Multiple Choice Questions

1. The Satellite cells in the Ganglia are:

   a. Macrophages;

   b. Supportive cells;

   c. Accessory cells;

   d. Pyramidal cells.

   (Answer: b)

2. Myelination in the Peripheral nerve is by:

   a. Astrocytes;

   b. Neuroglial cells;

   c. Oligodendrocytes;

   d. Schwann cells.

   (Answer: d)

3. Pseudounipolar neurons are seen in:

   a. Olfactory cells;

   b. Sensory ganglia;

   c. Cells of retina;

   d. Mesencephalic nucleus of Trigeminal nerve.

   (Answer: b)

4. Which of the following are Macroglial cells:

   a. Astrocytes;

   b. Oligodendrocytes;

   c. Ependymal cells;

   d. All of the above.

   (Answer: d)

Model Questions

Short Notes (5 Marks)

1. Differentiate between the microscopic picture of Sensory ganglion and Autonomic ganglion.

2. Histology of Peripheral nerve.

3. Draw a neat labeled diagram of microscopic picture of Optic nerve.

Chapter 14

SKIN AND ACCESSORY STRUCTURES

Objectives

1. The normal structure and functions of the thick Skin and thin Skin is important.
2. The skin appendages and their functions has to be known.

Definition: Skin is the largest and heaviest sensory organ of the body and forms $1/6^{th}$ of total body weight; it has a surface area of 18 sft.

Functions of Skin

1. Protects from trauma, uv rays & microorganisms;
2. Sensory perception: Through receptors for pain, temperature, touch and pressure.
3. Sweat glands regulate body temperature;
4. Epidermis helps in synthesis of vit. D from 7-dehydrocholesterol by action of uv-light.
5. It helps in the excretion of nitrogenous waste products and water;
6. The small arteriovenous anastomosis called as glomus are seen in the dermis which regulate blood pressure;
7. Skin helps in the absorption of chemicals, drugs and lipid soluble substances.
8. Skin is a store house of fat for glycogenolysis and cholesterol.

Histology of Skin

It consists of **outer epidermis** and **inner dermis.**

The two types of skin depending on the thickness of the epidermis are the thick or glabrous skin (palm and sole) which is non-hairy and thin skin (eyelids and almost all parts of the body) which is hairy.

Epidermis

Is made up of stratified squamous keratinized epithelium. It projects into the dermis through the epidermal ridges, it is avascular receives nutrition by diffusion.

The epidermis contains free nerve endings in the basal layers, keratinocytes, melanocytes, Langerhans cells, Merkel's cells, etc.

The epidermis is renewed every 15–30 days depending on the age, body, nutrition and other environmental/genetic factors. Epidermis has five layers:

1. **Stratum Corneum:** Is the superficial layer made up of keratin layer which consists of flat non-nucleated dead scaly cells with thick plasma membrane and cytoplasm filled with keratin. It's thin in thin skin and thick in thick skin. The cells are shed continuously.

2. **Stratum Lucidum:** Consists of a thin layer of flat eosinophilic dead cells with no nuclei, giving a homogenous glassy appearance. The cytoplasm has scleroproteins(keratin) derived from keratohyaline granules and tonofibrils.

3. **Stratum Granulosum:** It has 3–5 layers of flat fusiform cells having keratohyaline granules, the plasma membrane is covered with these granules, which provide a **"sealing effect"** against foreign substances.

4. **Stratum Spinosum:** This shows polygonal cells having cytoplasmic spine-like processes held together by desmosomes. This layer is well developed in areas of friction and pressure.

5. **Stratum Basale:** It has a single basal layer of columnar cells. Active mitosis takes place in this layer. Lower 2 layers are called as Malpighian layer.

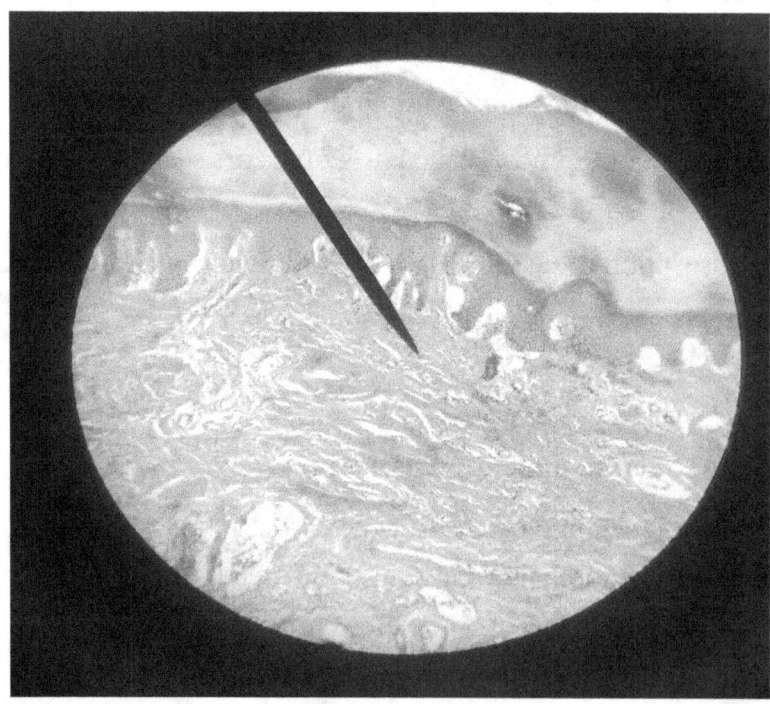

Histology of Thick Skin: 1

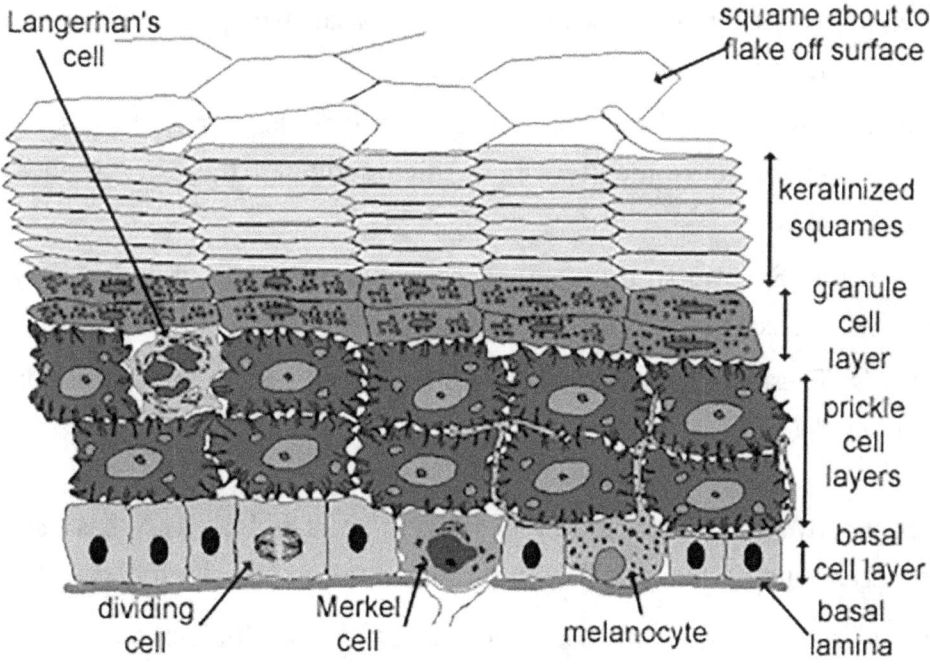

Cells Present in the Skin: 2

Thick Skin

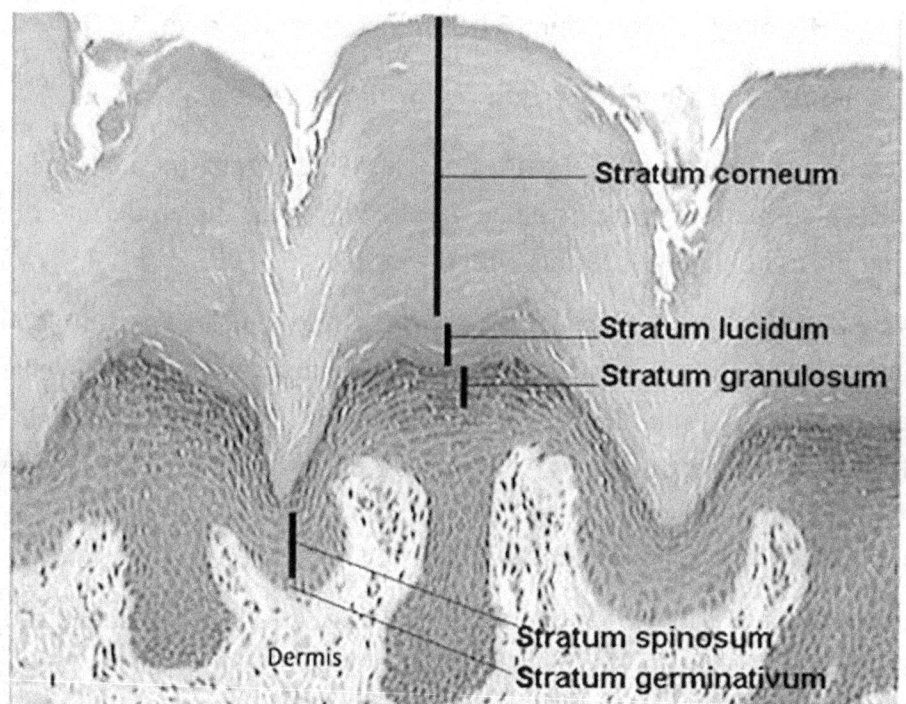

Thick Skin: 3

Histology of Thick Skin: 4 (for figure refer page no. 126)

Cells of Epidermis

- **Keratinocytes/Prickle Cells:** These are seen in the basal layer, produce KH granules/keratin (scleroprotein) and tonofibrils.

- **Melanocytes:** Derived from the neural crest cells in fetal life, seen in the basal layer, produce melanin pigments in melanosomes (tyrosinase) giving colour to the skin. Absence of tyrosinase gives rise to Albinism.

- **Langerhans Cells:** Seen in stratum spinosum, contain Bisbeck granules, they are antigen-presenting cells, protect against viral infections.

- **Merkel's Cells:** These are sensory cells (touch sensation) seen in the stratum basale.

Dermis

It consists of connective tissue with blood vessels, lymphatics and nerves, it has a superficial layer called *papillary layer* with dermal papillae and a deep *reticular layer* with fibrous tissue.

- The thin skin shows sweat glands, sebaceous glands, hair follicles and arrector pillorum.

- The thick skin shows many sweat glands and sensory nerve endings. It has no hair follicles and sebaceous glands.

Histology of Thin Skin: 5 (for figure refer page no. 126)

Histology of Thin Skin: 6 (for figure refer page no. 127)

Histology of Thin/Hairy Skin: 7 (for figure refer page no. 127)

Papillary Layer: Made up of loose CT with fibroblasts, macrophages, mast cells, etc. The CT projects into the epidermis as dermal papillae interlocking with the epidermal ridges. Collagen fibres/anchoring fibrils bind the epidermis with the dermis.

Reticular Layer: Contains type-1 collagen fibres which form the cleavage lines and elastic fibres for elasticity and firmness of the skin. Dermis also contains sweat glands, sebaceous glands, hair follicles and arrector pili muscles. Cutaneous receptors like Meissner's(touch) and Pacinian (pressure and vibrations) corpuscles are also present. Ruffini's corpuscle are sensitive to stretch.

Sebaceous Glands (Holocrine Gland)

It secrets sebum through a duct which opens into the hair follicle. It's a large group of rounded cells filled with fat droplets, therefore giving an empty look. Sebum is oily having antibacterial and antifungal actions; it contains lipids, cholesterol and esters.

It is controlled by testosterone in males and androgens in females.

Modified sebaceous glands are seen in the eye lids (Glands of Zeis, Moll and tarsal/Meibomian).

Sweat Glands/Sudoriferous Gland

It is a simple coiled tubular gland; its duct is lined by stratified cuboidal epithelium. Modified glands are the mammary and ceruminous glands.

There are 2 types:

- **Merocrine Gland:** Seen in dermis, small in size, tubule is lined by simple cuboidal cells(dark and light cells), ducts open into the skin surface, help in excretion and temperature control.

- **Apocrine Gland:** Seen in hypodermis, large in size, tubule is lined with simple cuboidal cells, ducts open into the hair follicle just above the sebaceous gland. Same functions as above.

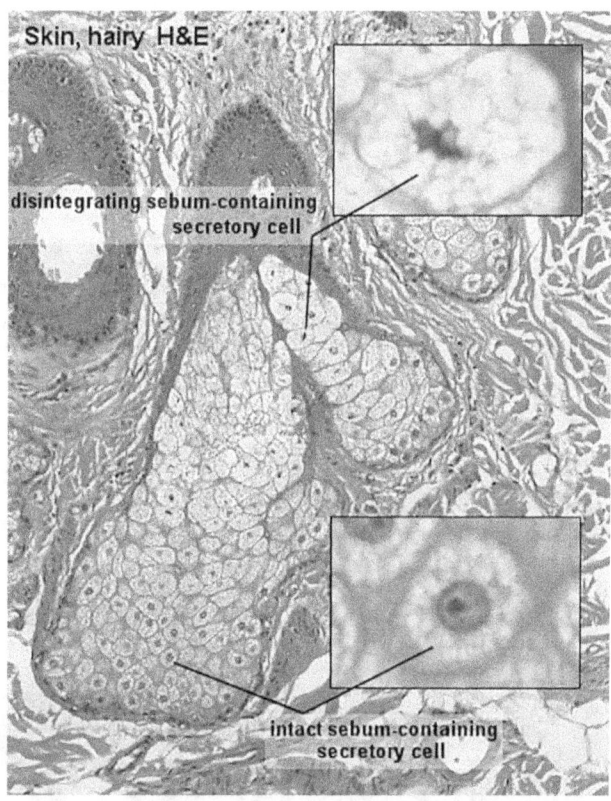

Histology of Sebaceous Gland: 8

Applied Aspects

1. Pale colour of the skin indicates Anaemia, yellow discoloration is seen in Jaundice, blue in cases of Cyanosis.

2. Loss of sensibility to touch is called as Anaesthesia and hypersensitivity to touch is called as Hyperaesthesia.

3. Depigmentation of skin is seen in Albinism and Vitiligo.

4. Full thickness and Split thickness skin grafting is done in excessive skin loss as in cases of burns.

Multiple Choice Questions

1. Which type of glands are Sebaceous glands:

    a. Merocrine;

    b. Holocrine;

    c. Apocrine;

    d. None of the above.

    (Answer: b)

2. Meissner's corpuscles are sensitive to:

    a. Temperature;

    b. Pressure;

    c. Pain;

    d. Touch.

    (Answer: d)

3. Merkel's Cells are sensory cells (touch sensation) seen in which stratum:

    a. Stratum basale;

    b. Stratum spinosum;

    c. Stratum granulosum;

    d. Stratum lucidum.

    (Answer: a)

4. Melanocytes are derived in fetal life from:

    a. Ectoderm;

    b. Neural crest cells;

    c. Mesoderm;

    d. Mesenchymal cells

    (Answer: b)

Model Questions

Short Notes (5 Marks)

1. Draw a neat labeled diagram of histology of Thick skin.

2. Describe the microscopic picture of all the layers of Hairy skin.

3. Describe the Skin Appendages.

Chapter 15

GLANDULAR TISSUE

Objectives

1. Classification of glands is necessary to understand their secretory function.

2. Exocrine and Endocrine glands, their structure and functions have to be known in detail.

Definition: Glands are secretory organs/cells which are derived from the epithelial tissue.

Classification of Glands

1. **Exocrine Glands:** These glands secrete out of the body by the ducts.

2. **Endocrine Glands:** Secrete within the body directly into the capillaries and require no ducts (ductless glands).

   1. **Exocrine Glands with Ducts:** Are of two types:

      a. **Unicellular Glands:** e.g. Goblet cells and secrete mucus as in small intestine.

      b. **Multicellular Glands:**

According to the Shape of the Glands

a. **Tubular Glands:** These can be straight (large intestine), coiled (sweat glands) or branched (stomach).

b. **Alveolar/Acinous:** In alveolar the gland is flask-shaped (palatine glands/mucus glands), in acinous the gland is rounded (pancreas, parotid glands/serous glands).

c. **Tubulo-alveolar:** A combination of both types. Mixed serous and mucus glands like the submandibular salivary glands.

According to the Ducts: Simple/Compound

a. **Simple Glands**: Unbranched and the secretion is conveyed to the surface, e.g. *Simple tubuloalveolar glands* – salivary glands, *Simple alveolar glands* – not seen in man.

b. **Compound Glands:** The duct branches into various types of glands, e.g. *compound tubular glands*- kidney, testis, *Compound tubulo-alveolar glands* – salivary glands, pancreas, *Compound alveolar glands* – mammary gland.

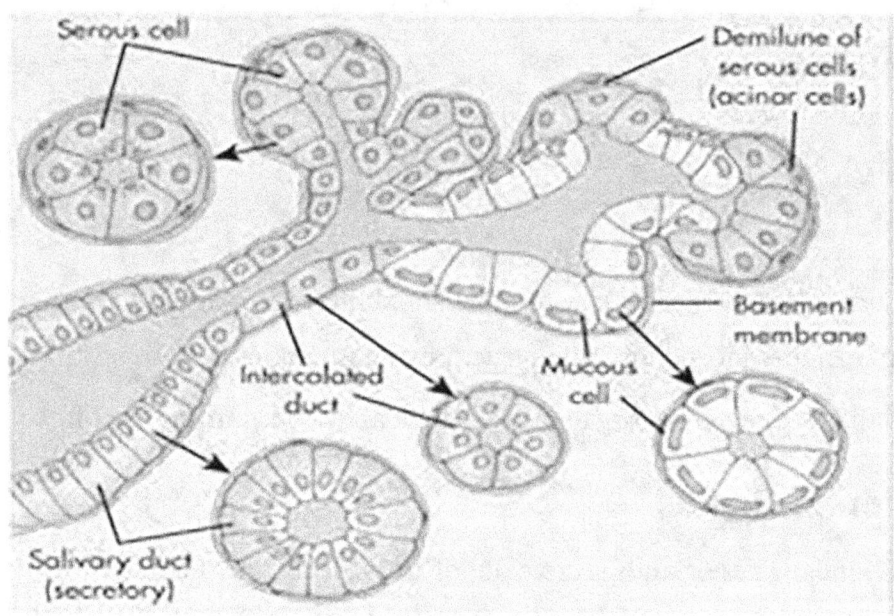

Acini and Duct System: 1

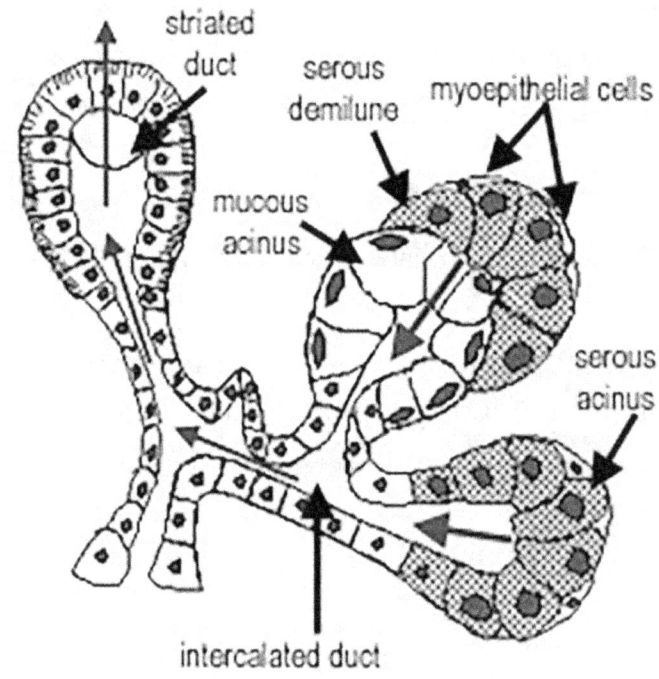

Serous and Mucous Acini: 2

According to the Manner of Secretion

a. **Holocrine:** The cells disintegrate and die to liberate the secretions, its a destructive process, e.g. Sebaceous glands.

b. **Apocrine:** The luminal part of the cell disintegrate, leaving the nucleus and the basal part from which the cell regenerates, e.g. mammary gland.

c. **Merocrine/Epicrine:** The secretion is discharged through the cell membrane without destruction of the cell. Most of the glands belong to this category.

According to the Development

a. **Ectodermal:** e.g. skin glands, mammary, pituitary, lacrimal and salivary glands.

b. **Mesodermal:** e.g. adrenal cortex, kidney, spleen.

c. **Endodermal:** e.g. thyroid, thymus, liver, pancreas.

According to the Nature of Secretions

a. **Mucous:** The secretion is thick, viscous and slimy, e.g. palatine glands, sublingual salivary gland.

b. **Serous:** The secretion is thin, watery, e.g. parotid salivary gland.

c. **Mixed:** Both mucous and serous are secreted, e.g. submandibular salivary gland.

Endocrine Glands

Cord and Clump Type: The endocrine glands secrete various hormones and are ductless glands, consisting of epithelial cells, reticular fibres and capillaries. The cords are irregular and store intracellular secretions, the secretion are expelled into the capillaries, e.g. adrenal gland, pancreas, testis, ovary.

Follicular Type: The cells clump together and secretion is by extracellular method, as seen in thyroid follicles.

Some glands are both exocrine and endocrine like the pancreas and testis.

Histology of Parotid Salivary Gland

It is a compound tubulo-acinar gland/racemose gland, purely a serous salivary gland, highly vascular with numerous blood vessels and well developed duct system.

It consists of numerous secretory end pieces called as serous acini, each acinous is rounded with narrow lumen and lined with pyramidal cells, each pyramidal cell shows basal striations with nucleus in the centre or slightly towards the base and the tip of the cells is pigmented due to zymogen granules, thereby taking a darker stain.

Histology of Parotid Gland: 3 (for figure refer page no. 128)

Histology of Parotid Gland: 4 (for figure refer page no. 128)

Histology of Parotid Gland: 5

The acini in the Parotid gland are arranged in groups called as lobules which are separated by the interlobular connective tissue with blood vessels and lymphatics.

Each acinous has myoepithelial cell between the cell membrane and basal lamina. These are contractile units of the gland which help to expel the secretions.

The connective tissue which supports the parenchyma forms the stroma, the parenchyma consists of the acini and the ducts. The stroma consists of the capsule, interlobar, interlobular and intralobular CT septae.

The CT septae contain blood vessels, nerves, lymphatics and interlobular ducts.

The *main excretory duct* divides into *interlobar ducts* then into *interlobular ducts* which again divide into *intralobular ducts/striated ducts, the basal striations in the ducts are due to vertical infoldings of the plasma membrane and vertical arrangement of the* mitochondria.

The small *intercalated ducts* which opens into the acini also show the myoepithelial cells.

The main large excretory duct is lined by *stratified columnar epithelium*, the other ducts are lined with *simple columnar epithelium* and the intercalated ducts are lined with *simple cuboidal epithelium*.

The cells lining the ducts help to regulate the water and electrolytes present in the saliva making it **hypotonic**, they also show **Ig A.**

Histology of Submandibular Gland

It is a mixed type of salivary gland containing both serous and mucous acini.

Mucous acinous is larger in size, with large lumen, it is lined with flat cells, containing mucoid substance which pushes the nucleus towards the base making it flat. Due to the mucoid secretion it takes light pink stain giving it an empty look.

The mucous secretions keep the mouth moist, provides protection and lubrication, enzymes like amylase and Ig A are also present.

Apart from the mucous acini, the gland shows **serous demilunes**, here, the mucous acinous is covered by a crescent/half-moon shaped serous acinous. Such demilunes are also seen in **sublingual gland** which is purely a mucous gland.

Histology of Submandibular Gland: 6 (for figure refer page no. 129)

Histology of Submandibular Gland: 7 (for figure refer page no. 129)

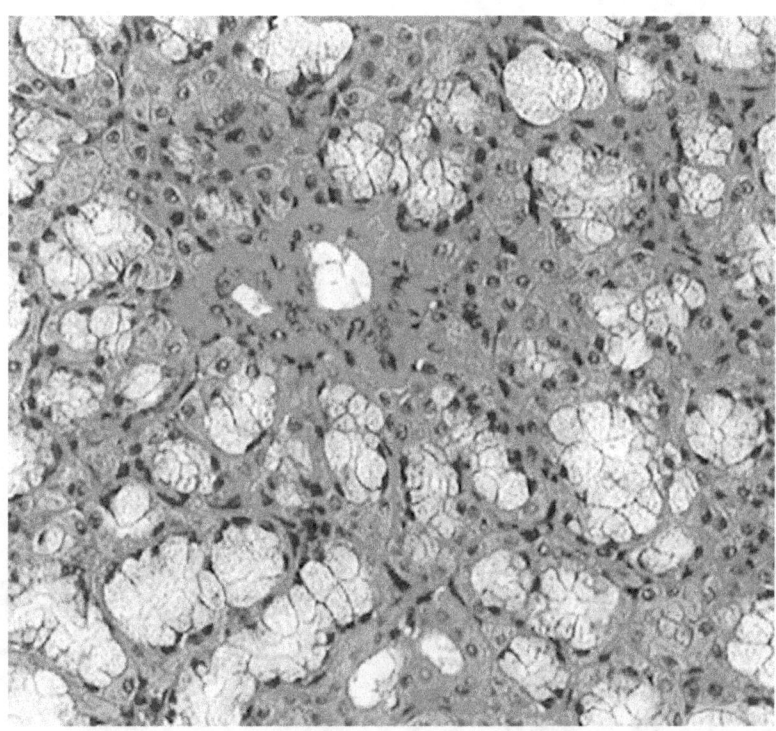

Histology of Submandibular Gland: 8

Applied Aspects

1. Enlargement of the Parotid salivary gland is seen in viral infections like Mumps.

2. Presence of stones or calculi in the duct system of the salivary glands can be detected by procedure known as Sialography.

Multiple Choice Questions

1. The Parotid gland consists of predominantly of which type of acini:

    a. Mucous acini;

    b. Serous acini;

    c. Mixed acini,

    d. None of the above.

    (Answer:b)

2. Pancreas is which type of gland:

    a. Exocrine;

    b. Endocrine;

    c. Both exocrine and endocrine;

    d. None of the above.

    (Answer: c)

3. The intercalated ducts are lined with:

    a. Simple cuboidal epithelium;

    b. Simple columnar epithelium;

    c. Simple squamous epithelium;

    d. None of the above.

    (Answer: a)

Model Questions

Short Notes (5 Marks)

1. Histology of Parotid gland.
2. Microscopic picture of Submandibular gland.

Chapter 16

PLACENTA AND UMBILICAL CORD

Objectives

1. Structure and functions of Placenta is important.
2. Anomalies of Placenta.
3. Structure of Umbilical cord.

Development of Placenta

At the beginning of the **3rd. week,** the trophoblast forms **the primary villi** consisting of inner *cytotrophoblastic core* and an *outer syncytial layer.* The mesodermal core grows towards the decidua, forming the loose mesenchymal tissue in its central core, thus, this forms the **secondary chorionic villi.** These cover the entire chorionic sac, some of the cells go to form the blood cells and capillaries, now the villi are called as **tertiary chorionic villi/definitive placental villi.**

The capillaries of the mesoderm, develop in the chorionic plate and in the connecting stalk, thus, connecting the placenta with the embryo.

At the **4th. week** the heart begins to beat, and the villus system begins to supply nutrients and oxygen to the embryo. The cytotrophoblast forms a shell around the syncytiotrophoblast, the villi attached to this shell are called as *anchoring villi/stem chorionic villi.* The villi that grow from the sides of the stem villi are called as *terminal villi/branch chorionic villi. It is through this that the exchange of nutrients and gases takes place.*

At **8th. week** the entire chorionic sac is covered by chorionic villi, as the sac grows it gets compressed by the outer decidua capsularis, and that part gets degenerated producing the avascular area called as *chorionic laeve.*

The villi related to the decidua basalis increase in number and branch profusely to form the *chorionic frondosum.* Thus, at the embryonic pole is the chorionic frondosum, and at the abembryonic pole is the chorionic laeve.

Functions of Placenta

◆   Protection;

◆   Exchange of nutients, electrolytes like aminoacids, vitamins, fattyacids, etc.

◆   Respiration: Exchange of gases like oxygen (fetus takes 20–30 ml of oxygen/min.);

◆   Excretion of carbon dioxide and waste products;

◆   *Hormone production:* syncytiotrophoblast of placenta produces progesterone, estriol, human chorionic gnadotropins (hcg), placental lactogen, etc.

◆   Transmission of maternal IgG antibodies.

◆   Drugs can cross the placental barrier by simple diffusion;

◆   Infections like rubella, measles, polio viruses can pass through the placental barrier.

Structure of Placenta

The placenta consists of two components at 16 weeks:

◆   *Fetal Part:* develops from the chorionic sac;

◆   *Maternal Part:* Is derived from the ***endometrium / decidua basalis.*** At fetal side is the ***chorionic plate*** and at the maternal side is the ***decidual plate,*** inbetween these plates is the intervillous space containing the maternal blood. The shape of placenta is ***circular / discoid shape.*** *Irregular areas called as* ***cotyledons*** *are seen towards the fetal side and the* ***placental septum*** *is seen towards the maternal side.*

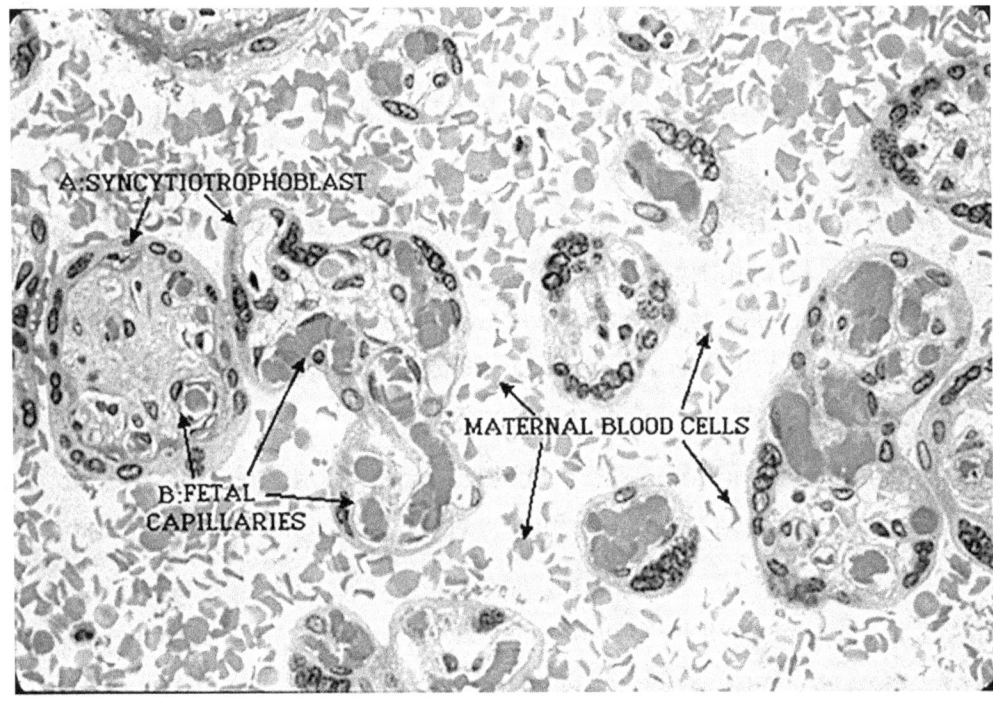

Placenta: 1

Placenta: 2 (for figure refer page no. 130)

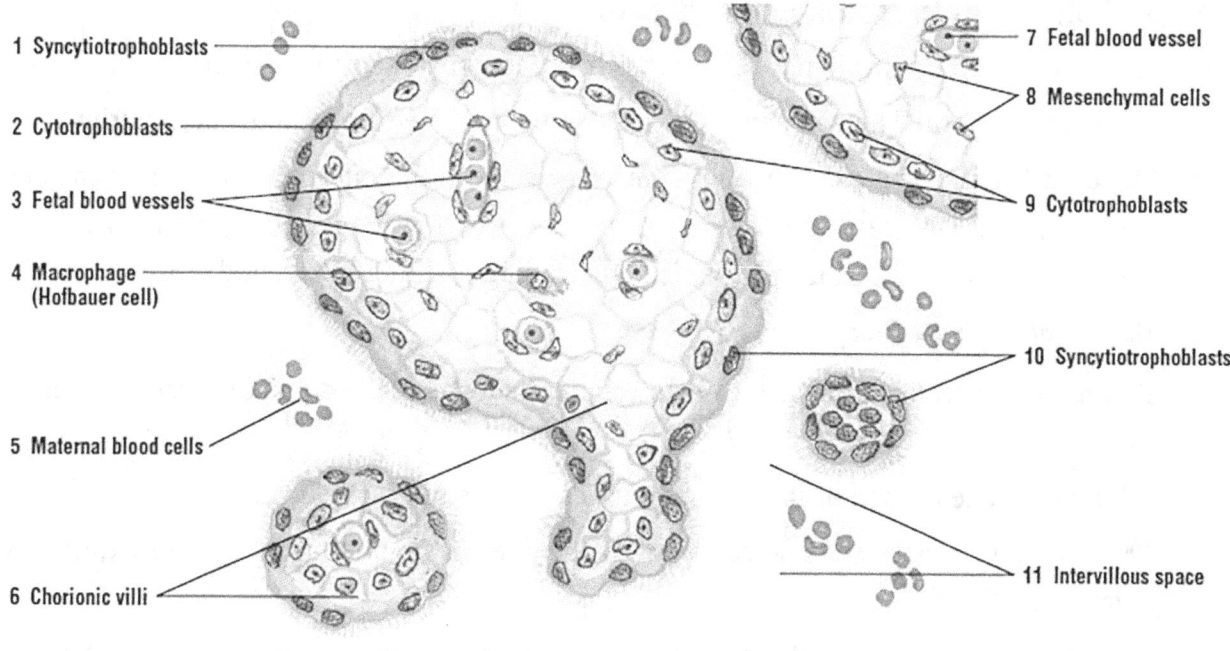

1 Syncytiotrophoblasts
2 Cytotrophoblasts
3 Fetal blood vessels
4 Macrophage (Hofbauer cell)
5 Maternal blood cells
6 Chorionic villi
7 Fetal blood vessel
8 Mesenchymal cells
9 Cytotrophoblasts
10 Syncytiotrophoblasts
11 Intervillous space

Placenta: 3

Placenta: 4 (for figure refer page no. 130)

Placental Barrier and Circulation

The chorionic villi provide a very thin layer for the exchange of materials called as *placental barrier/placental membrane*, which is between the fetal and maternal circulations. This is made up of *four layers:*

1. Endothelial lining of fetal vessels;
2. Connective tissue in the villus;
3. Cytotrophoblastic layer and
4. Syncytio-trophoblastic layer.

PLACENTAL CIRCULATION: The deoxygenated blood leaves the fetus through the umbilical arteries, which divide into various chorionic arteries in the choronic plate.

This arterio-venous system communicates with the maternal blood, and provides a large area for exchange of nutrients/gases. All the veins join to form the umbilical vein, which carry oxygenated blood to the fetus. The blood enters through the spiral arteries into the decidua basalis, through the chorionic plate. The exchange of materials takes place in the inter-villus spaces.

Anomalies of Placenta

1. **Depending on Its Attachment to the Uterus**

    a. **Placenta Accreta:** Chorionic villi are attached to the myometrium of uterus.

    b. **Placenta Percreta:** The villi penetrate through the myometrium and the perimetrium.

    c. **Placenta Previa:** The blastocyst implants very close to the internal os of uterus causing haemorrhage. This can occur either in the upper or lower uterine segments. In lower uterine segment it can cause severe bleeding leading to difficulty in child birth.

    Degrees of Placenta Praevia

    1st.degree: Placenta is attached to the lower uterine segment but does not cover the internal os.

    2nd.degree: The margin of the placenta just covers the internal os.

    3rd.degree: The edge of the placenta covers the internal os, but it does not cause difficulty in labour.

    4th.degree: Placenta completely covers the internal os and occludes the os, causing obstructed labour.

2. **Depending on Shape of Placenta**

    a. **Bidiscoidal Shape:** Consists of two discoid-shaped placentas.

    b. **Diffuse Shape:** Chorionic villi are seen all around the blastocyst, placenta is thin and irregular.

    c. **Lobed:** The placenta is divided into various lobes.

    d. **Placenta Succenturiata:** A small part of the placenta is separated from the rest of it.

    e. **Fenestrated:** There's a hole in the placenta.

    f. **Circumvallate:** The edges are covered with circular fold of decidua.

Histology of Umbilical Cord

The umbilical cord is a helical and tubular blood conduit connecting the foetus to the placenta. The umbilical cord achieves its final form by the 12th week of gestation and normally contains two arteries and a single vein. The umbilical cord is mostly made up of connective tissue known as Wharton's Jelly and has relatively few cells and is surrounded by amnion. The umbilical vessels transport blood to and from the placenta, where exchange between the mother and fetus takes place. It has an average length of 50–60 cms. Very long cords may be associated with prolapse, looping of the cord around the foetal neck, entanglement, distress and foetal death. On the other hand very short cords may lead to delayed foetal descent, premature placental separation, growth retardation, congenital abnormalities, foetal distress and fetal death.

Cross Section of Umbilical Cord: 5 (for figure refer page no. 131)

Cross Section of Umbilical Cord: 6 (for figure refer page no. 131)

Multiple Choice Questions

1. The functions of Placenta include the following except:

    a. Protection;

    b. Exchange of nutrients,

    c. Exchange of gases like oxygen ;

    d. Does not transmit maternal IgG antibodies.

    (Answer: d)

2. The umbilical cord has:

    a. 2 arteries and 1 vein;

    b. 2 arteries and 2 veins;

    c. 1artery and 2 veins;

    d. 1 artery and 1 vein.

    (Answer: a)

Model Questions

Short Notes (5 Marks)

1. Describe the microscopic structure of Placenta.

2. Histology of umbilical cord.

3. Write the functions of Placenta.

4. Write the development and anomalies of placenta.

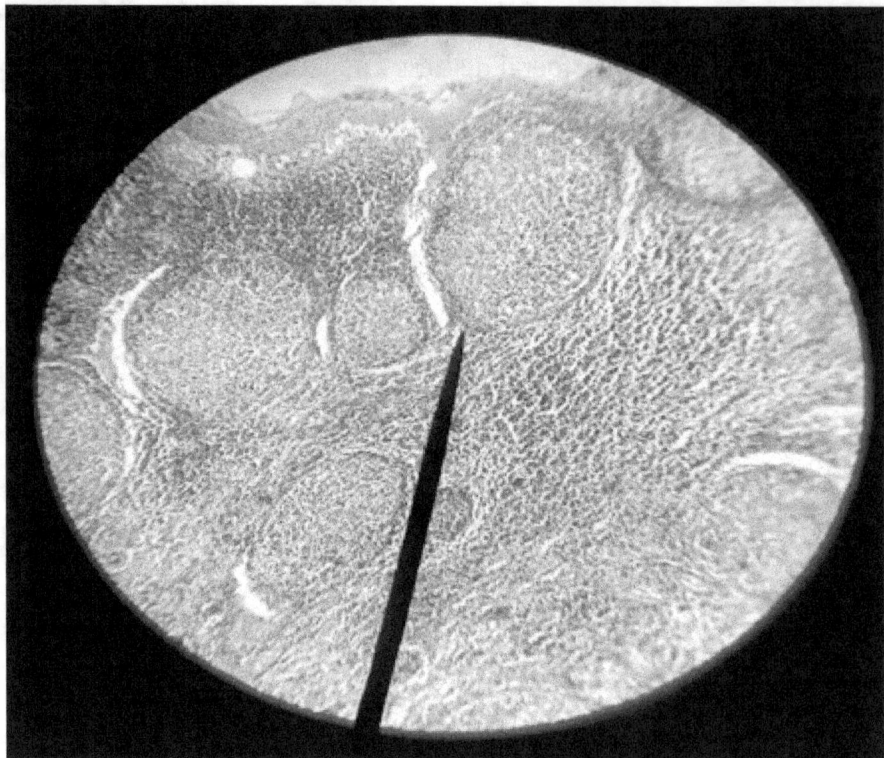

Histology of Lymph Node: 4

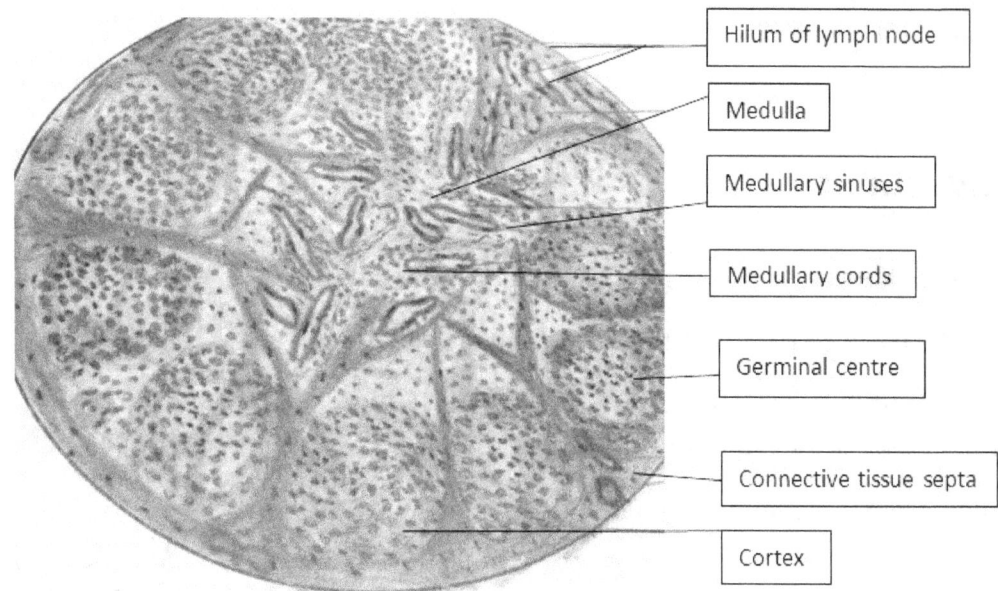

Lymph Node: 6

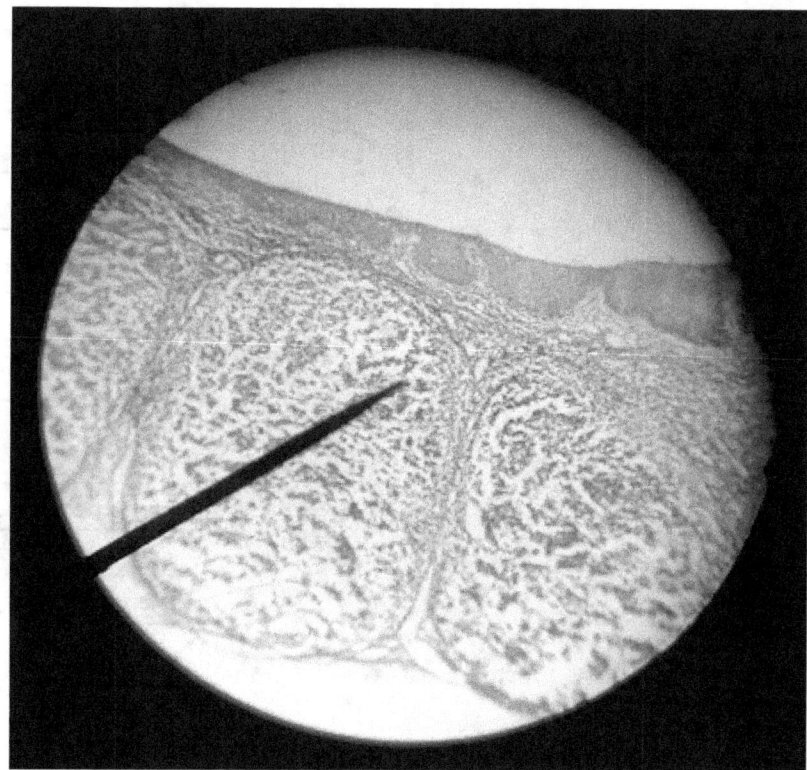

Histology of Palatine Tonsil: 7

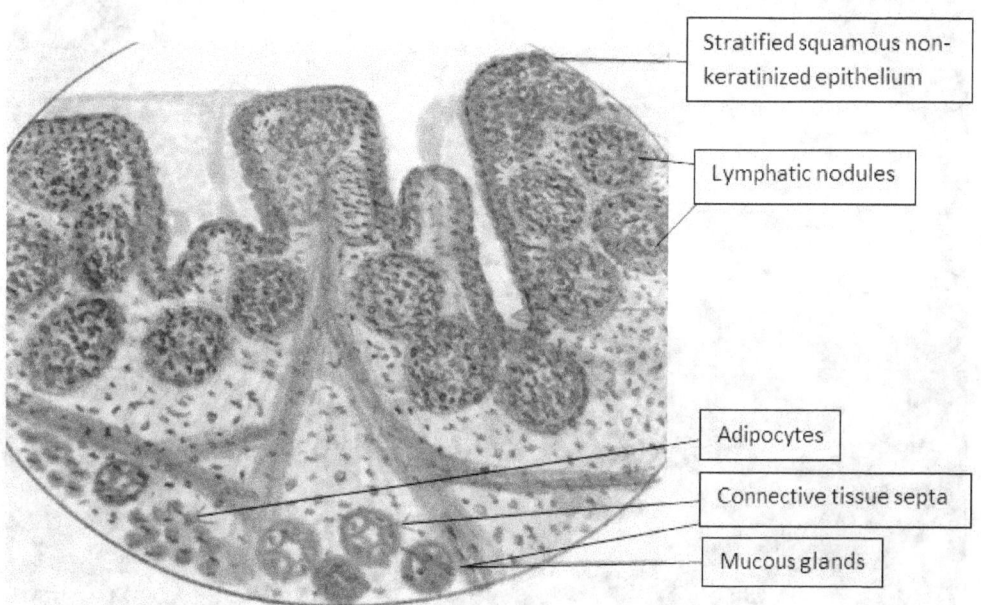

Histology of Palatine Tonsil: 9

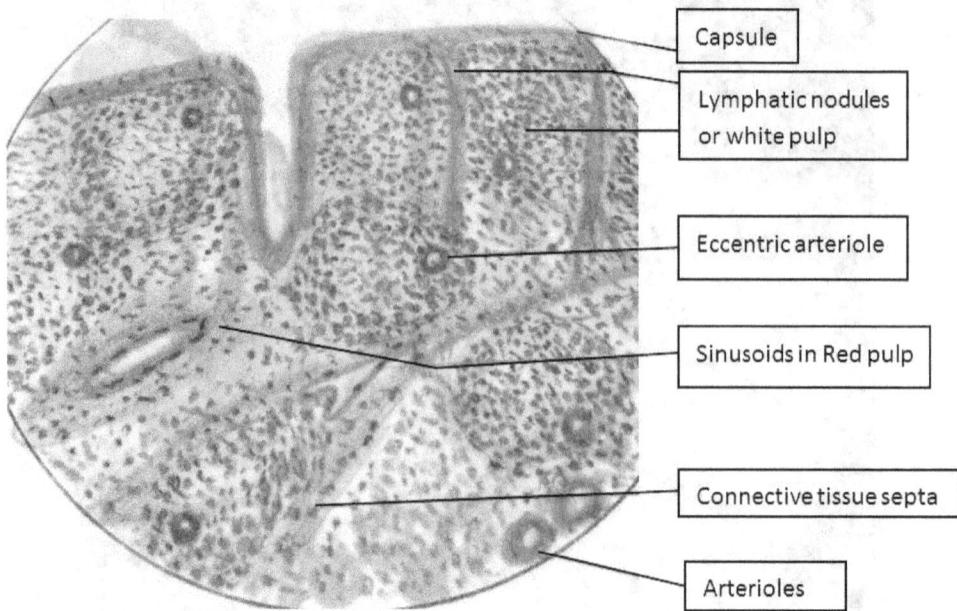

	Capsule
	Lymphatic nodules or white pulp
	Eccentric arteriole
	Sinusoids in Red pulp
	Connective tissue septa
	Arterioles

Histology of Spleen: 11

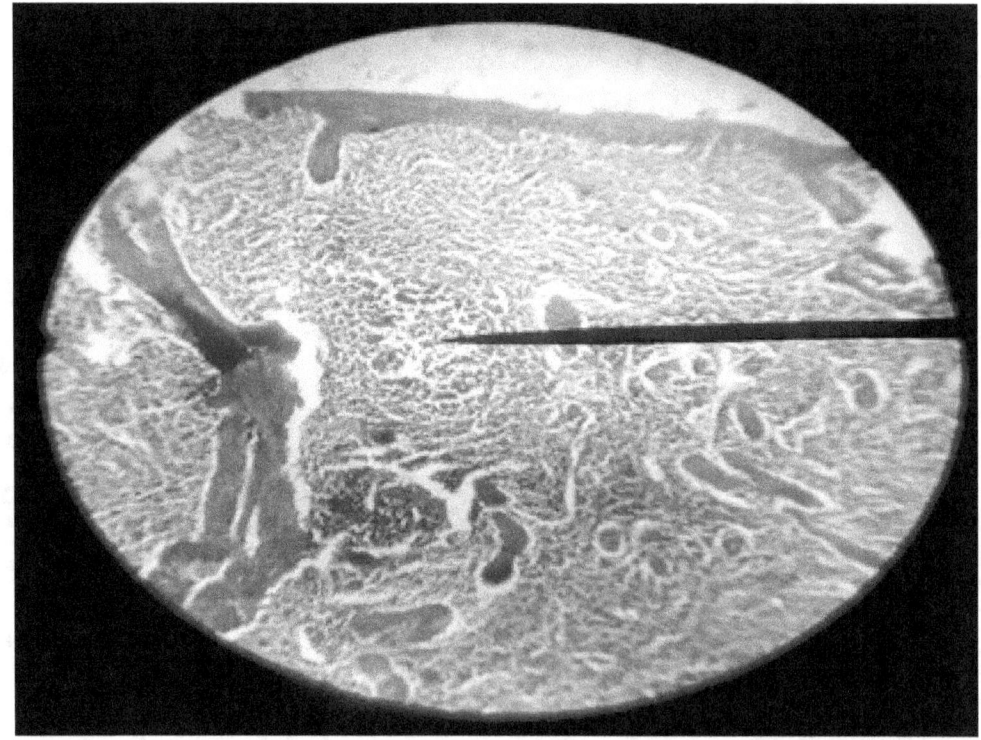

Histology of Spleen: 13

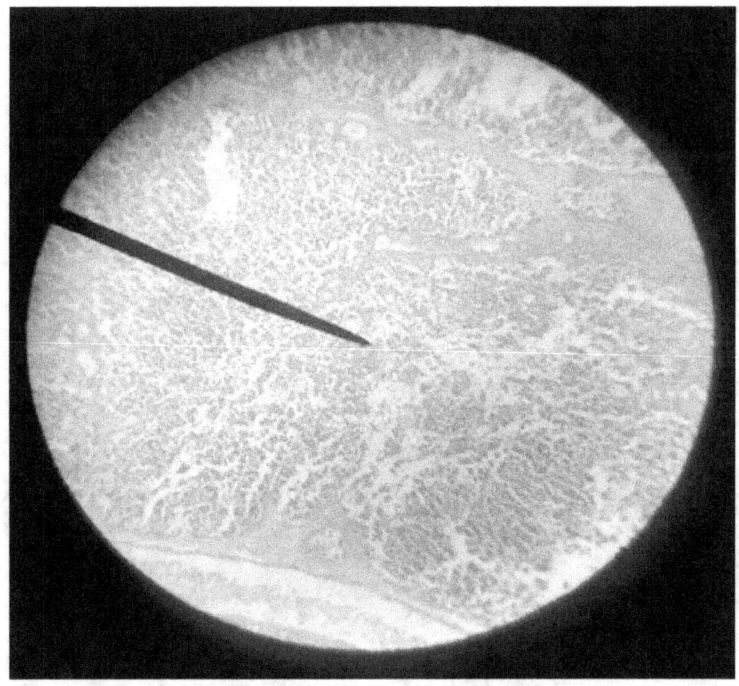

Histology of Thymus: 14

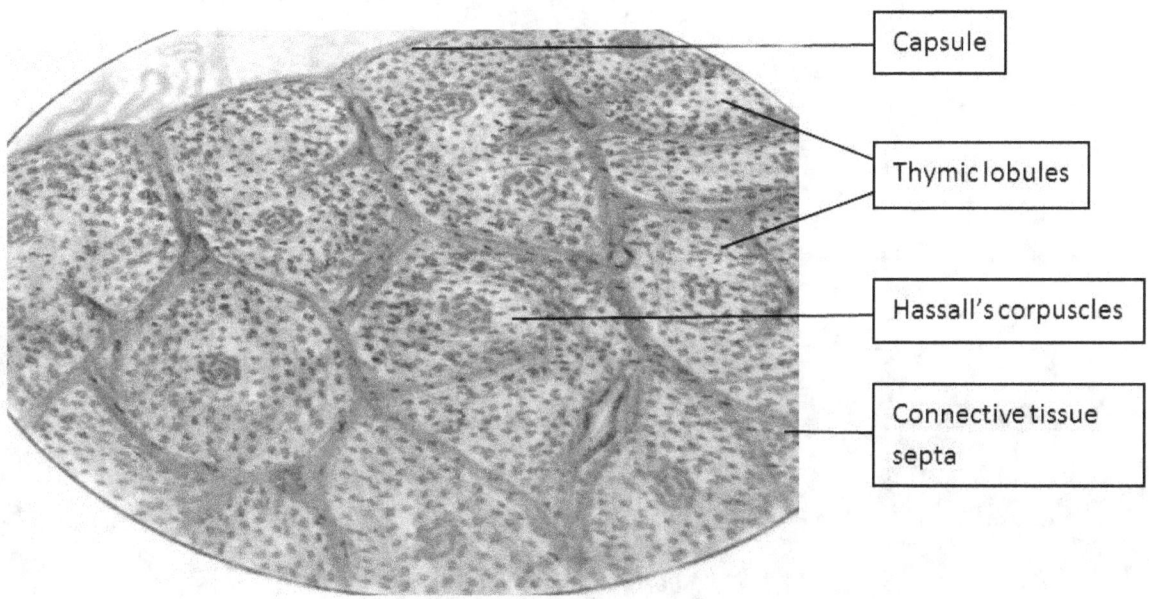

Histology of Thymus: 16

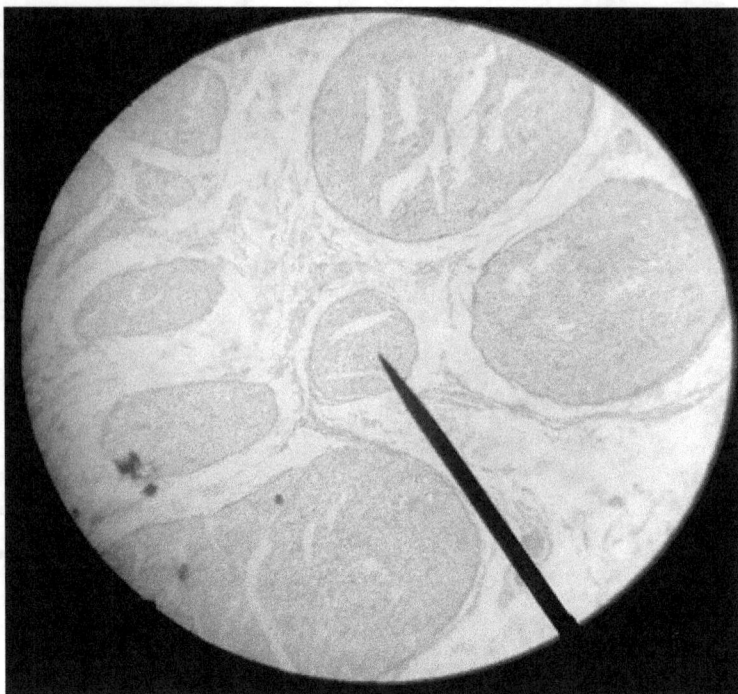

Histology of Peripheral Nerve: 5

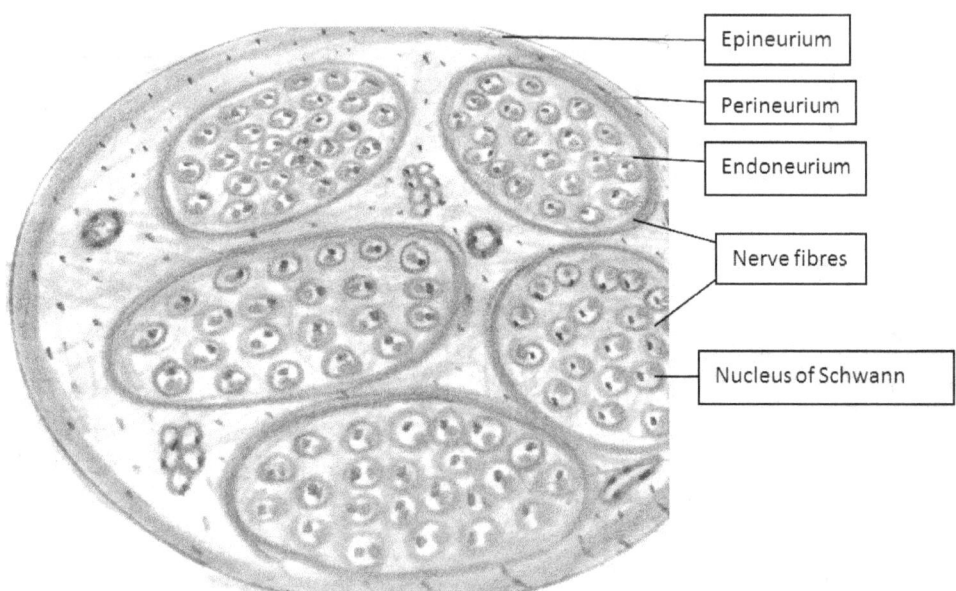

Epineurium

Perineurium

Endoneurium

Nerve fibres

Nucleus of Schwann

Peripheral Nerve: 6

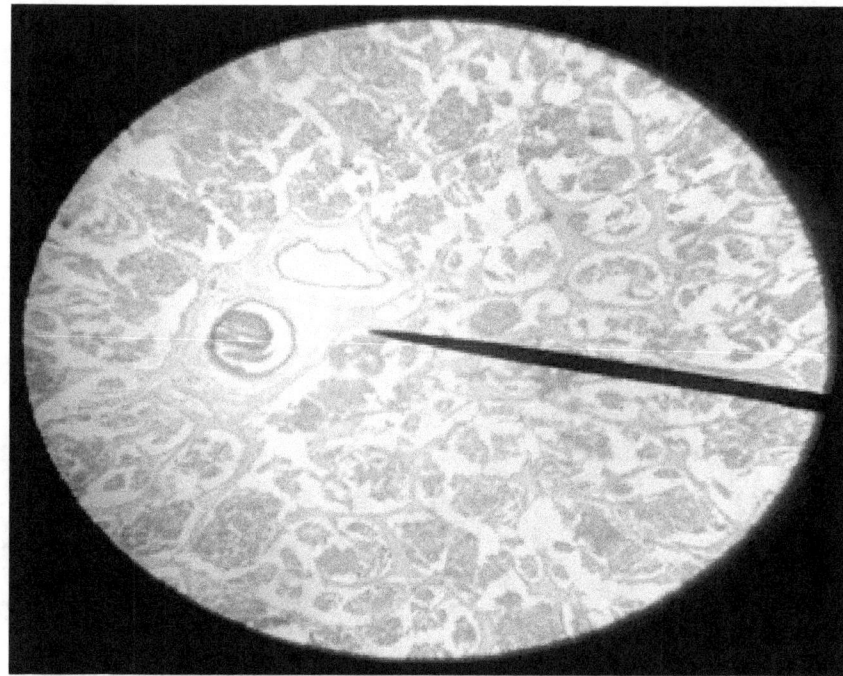

Histology of Optic Nerve: 10

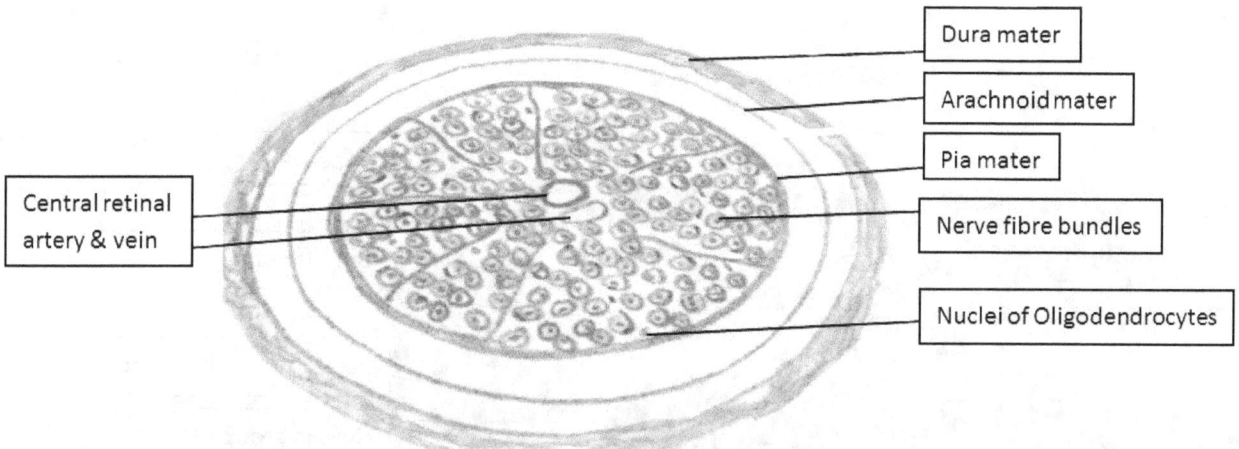

Optic Nerve: 12

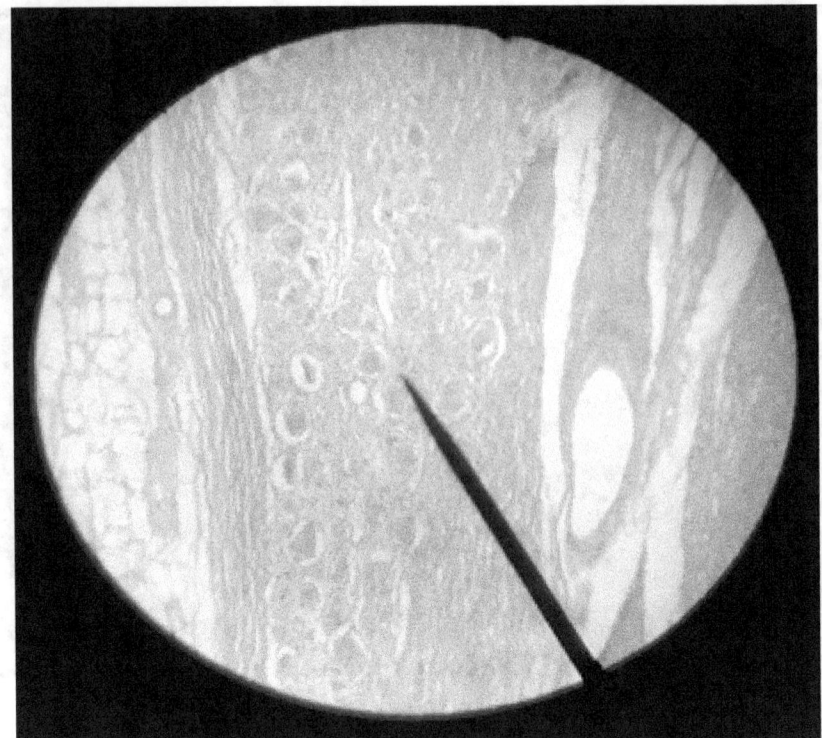

Sensory Ganglion: 13

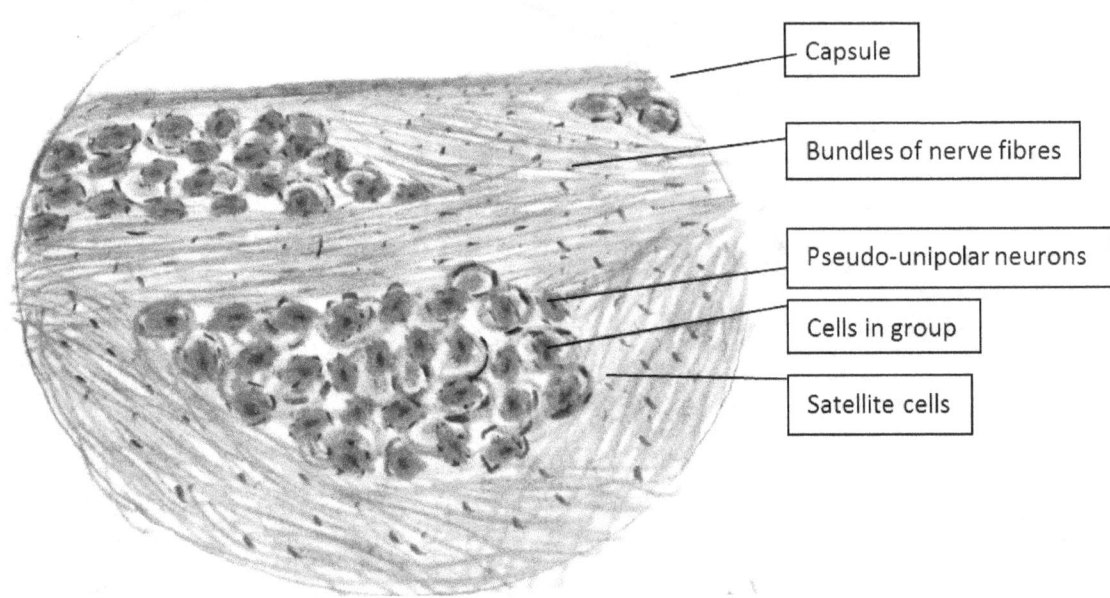

Capsule

Bundles of nerve fibres

Pseudo-unipolar neurons

Cells in group

Satellite cells

Sensory Ganglion: 14

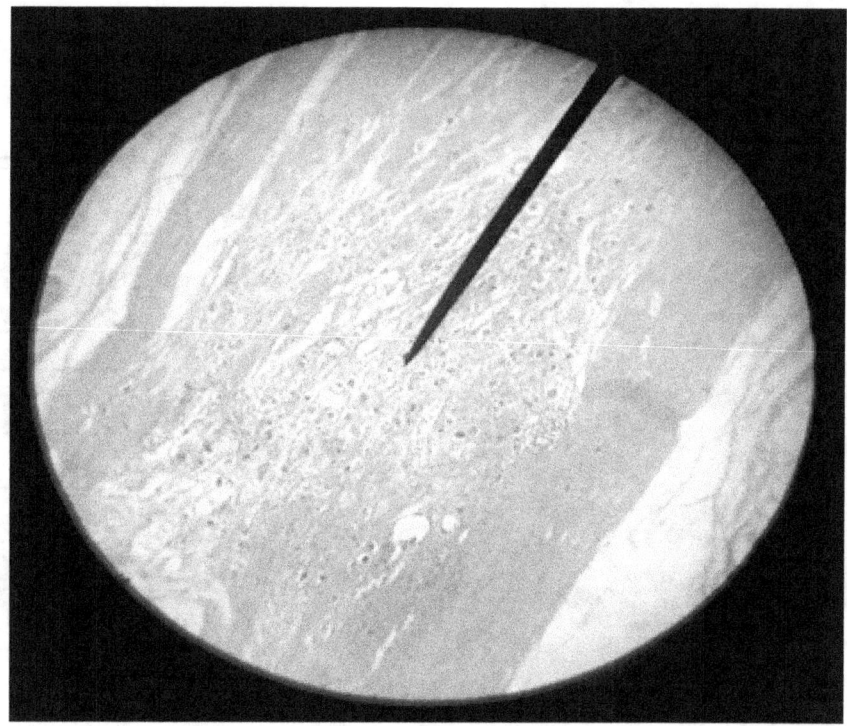

Autonomic Ganglion: 16

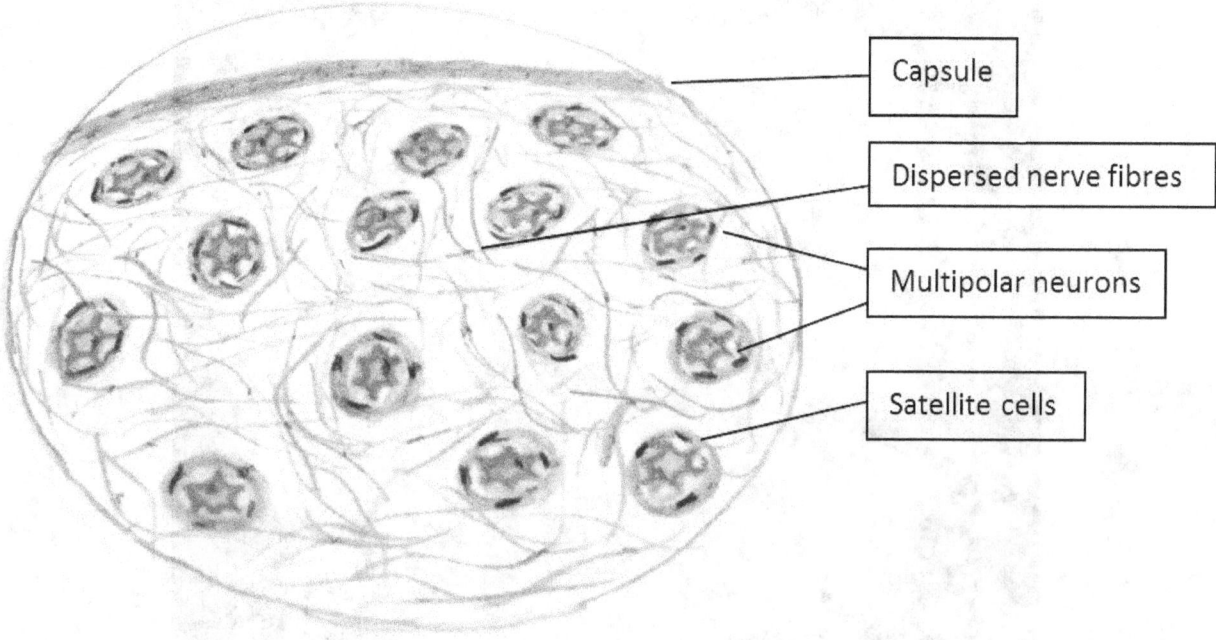

Capsule

Dispersed nerve fibres

Multipolar neurons

Satellite cells

Autonomic Ganglion: 17

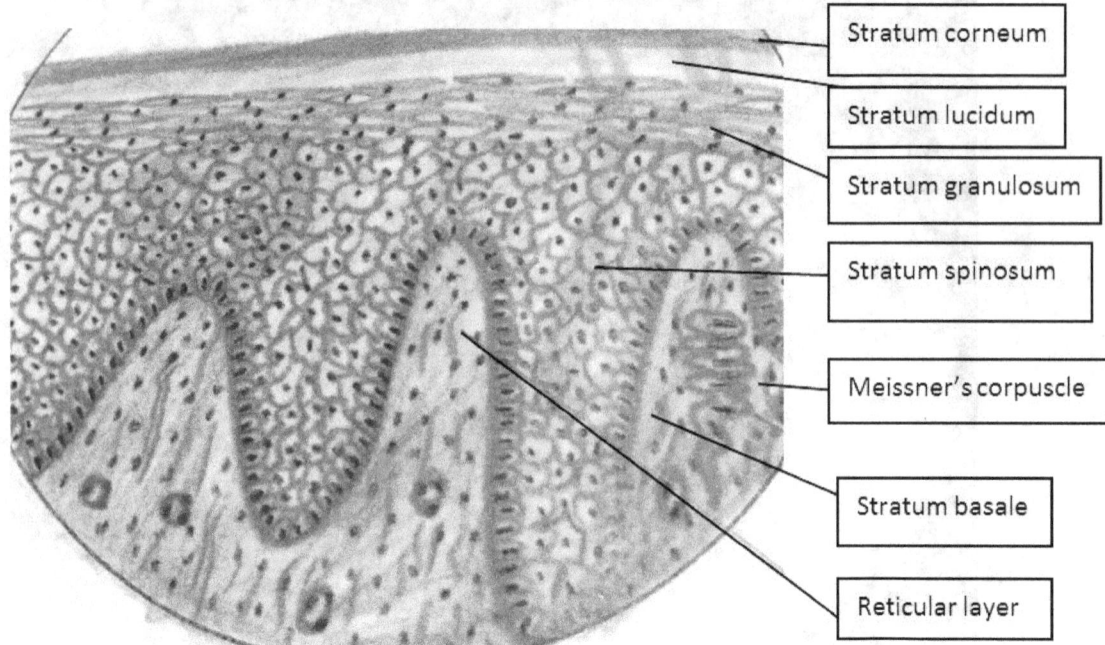

Stratum corneum

Stratum lucidum

Stratum granulosum

Stratum spinosum

Meissner's corpuscle

Stratum basale

Reticular layer

Histology of Thick Skin: 4

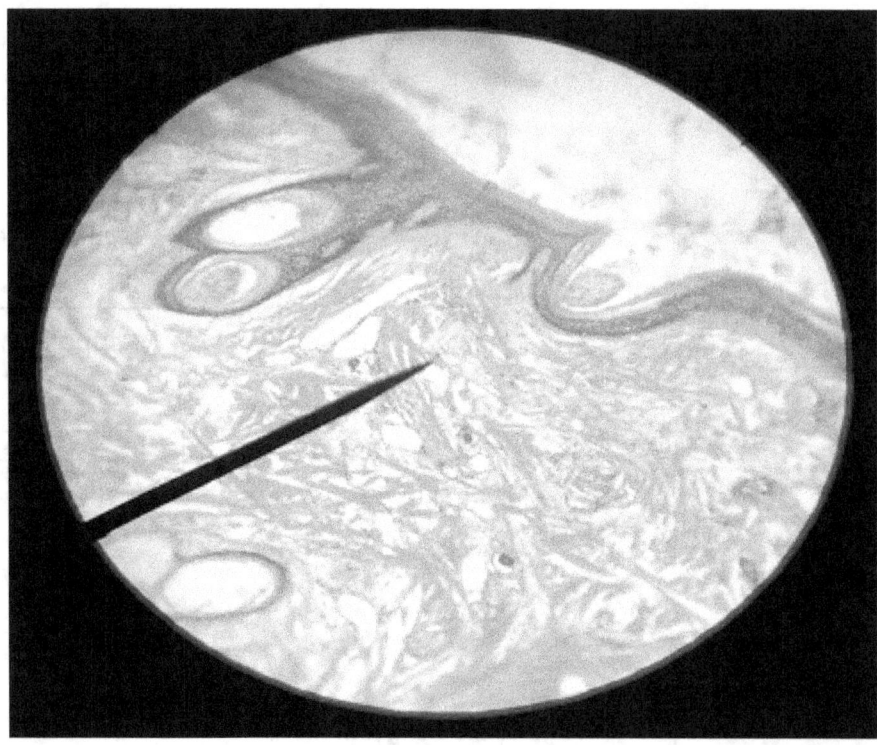

Histology of Thin Skin: 5

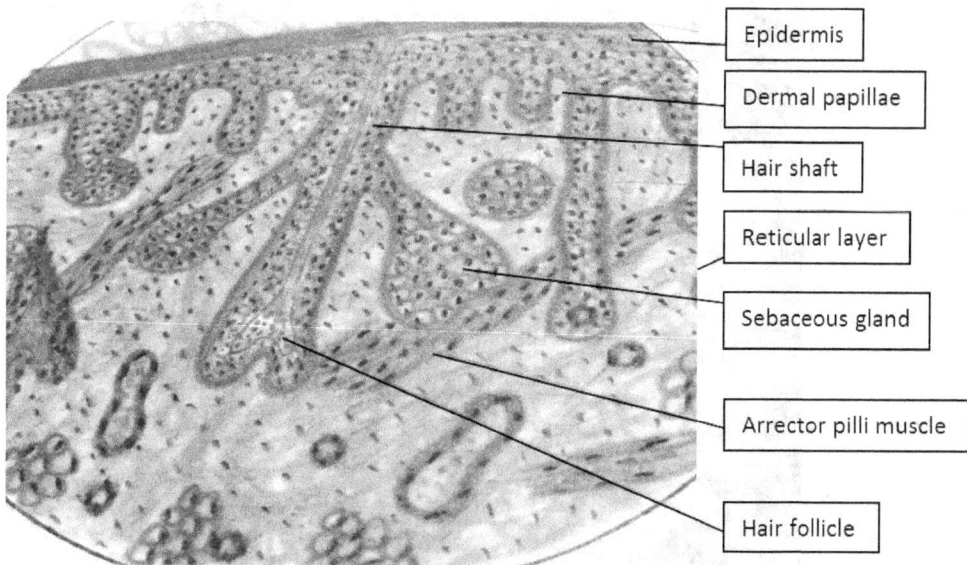

- Epidermis
- Dermal papillae
- Hair shaft
- Reticular layer
- Sebaceous gland
- Arrector pilli muscle
- Hair follicle

Histology of Thin/Hairy Skin: 7

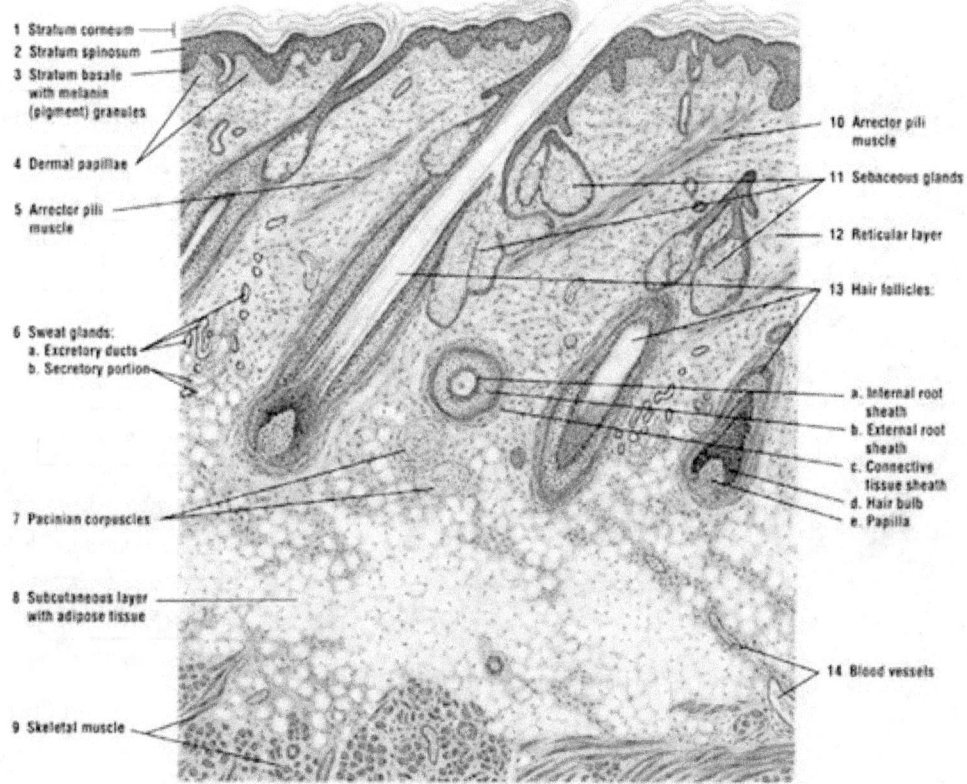

1 Stratum corneum
2 Stratum spinosum
3 Stratum basale with melanin (pigment) granules
4 Dermal papillae
5 Arrector pili muscle
6 Sweat glands:
   a. Excretory ducts
   b. Secretory portion
7 Pacinian corpuscles
8 Subcutaneous layer with adipose tissue
9 Skeletal muscle

10 Arrector pili muscle
11 Sebaceous glands
12 Reticular layer
13 Hair follicles:
   a. Internal root sheath
   b. External root sheath
   c. Connective tissue sheath
   d. Hair bulb
   e. Papilla
14 Blood vessels

Histology of Thin Skin: 6

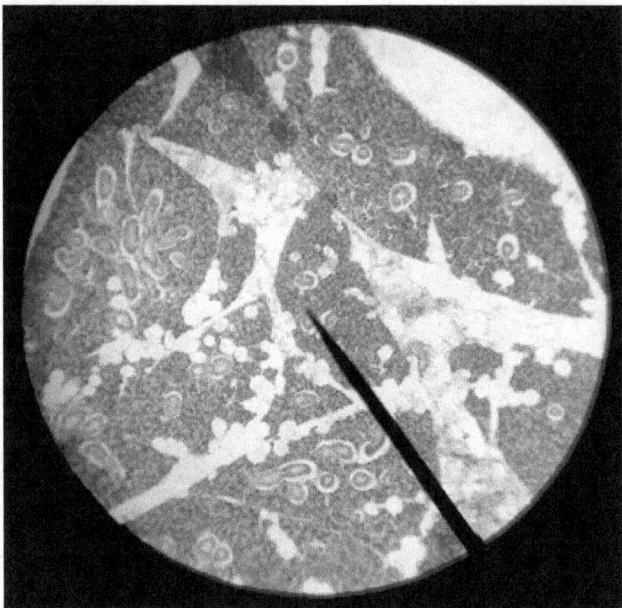

Histology of Parotid Gland: 3

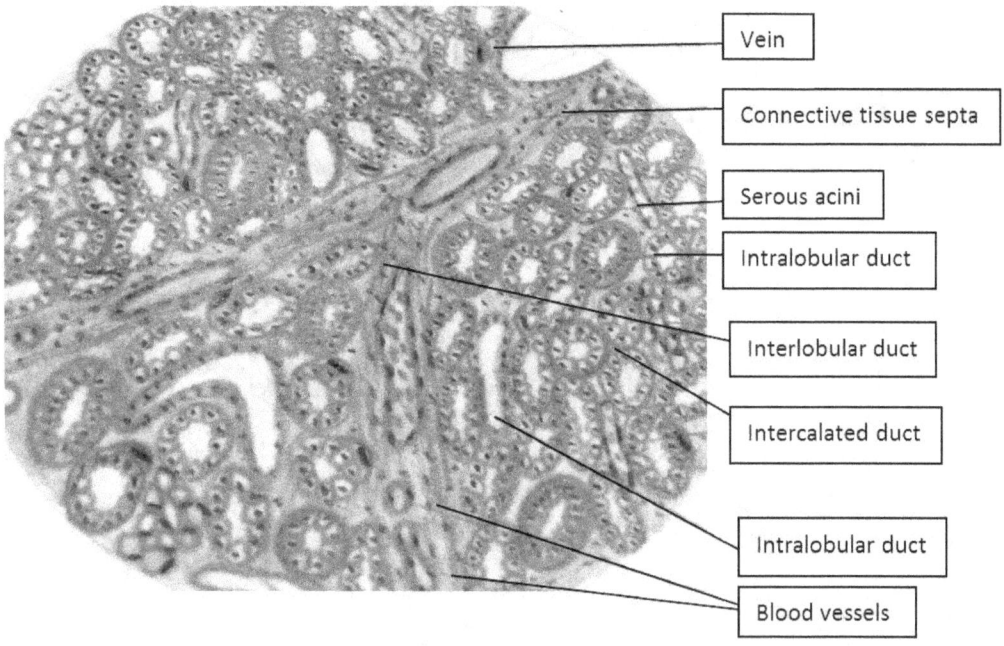

Histology of Parotid Gland: 4

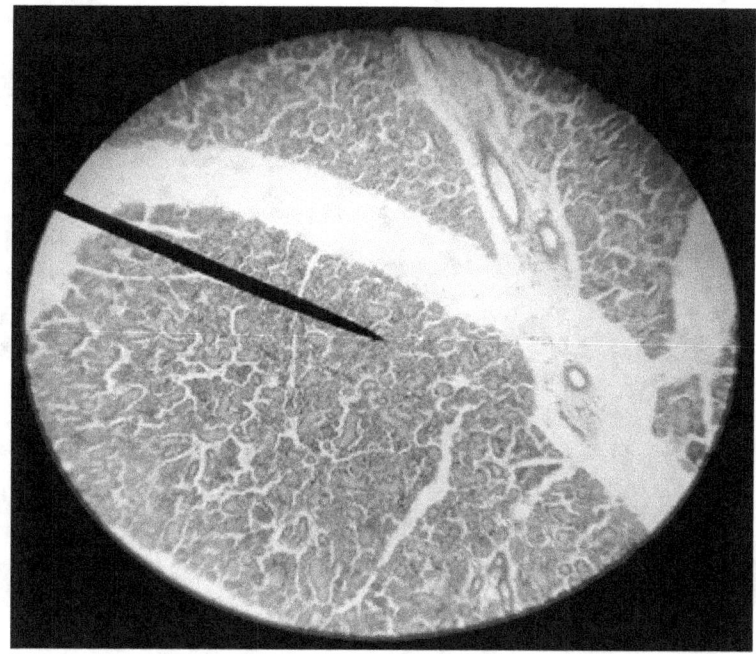

Histology of Submandibular Gland: 6

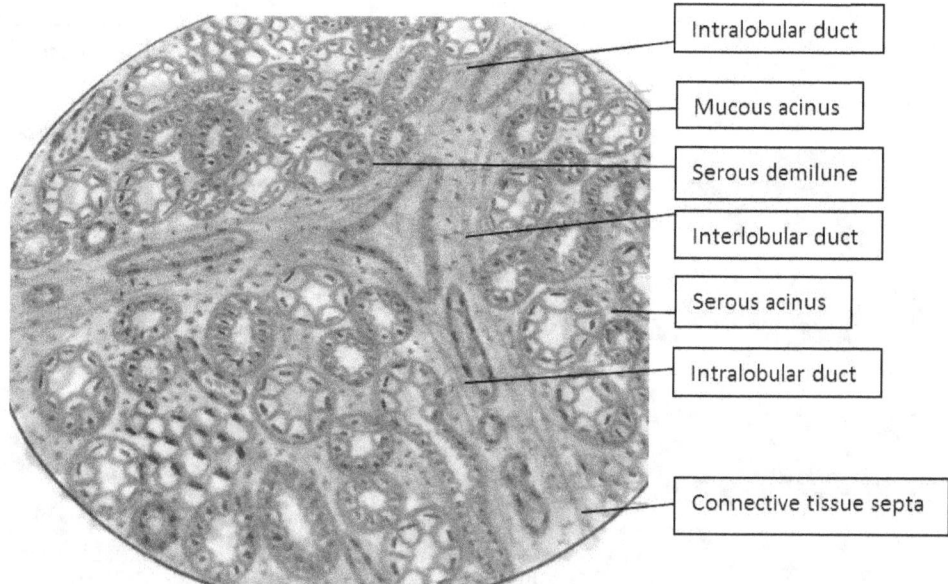

Histology of Submandibular Gland: 7

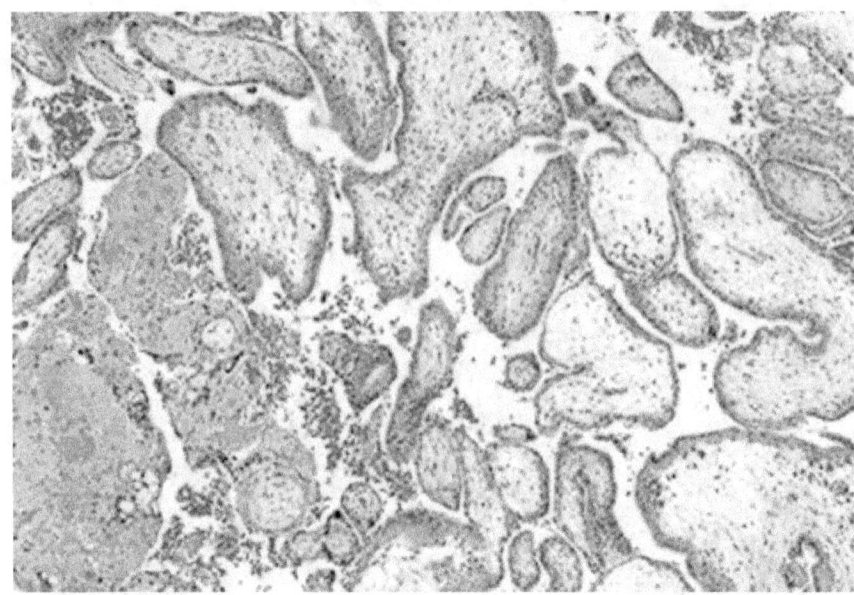

Placenta: 2

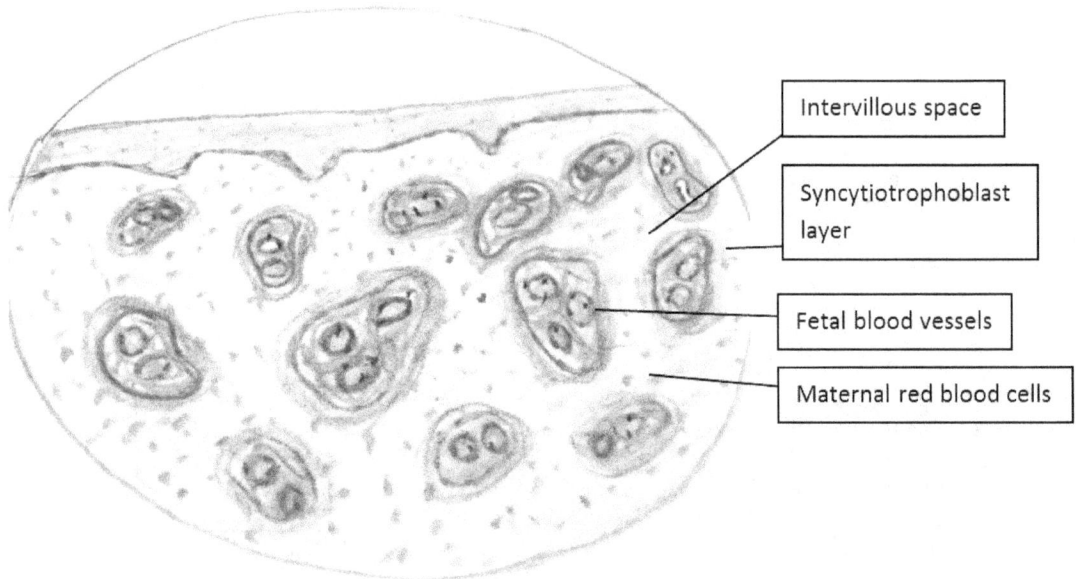

Placenta: 4

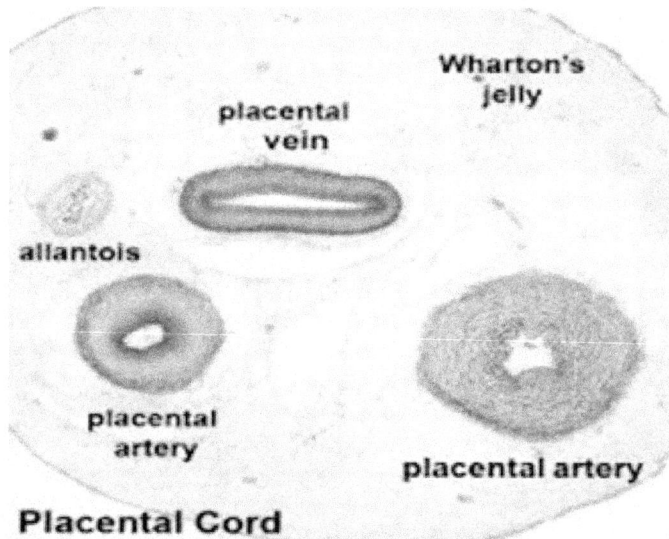

Cross Section of Umbilical Cord: 5

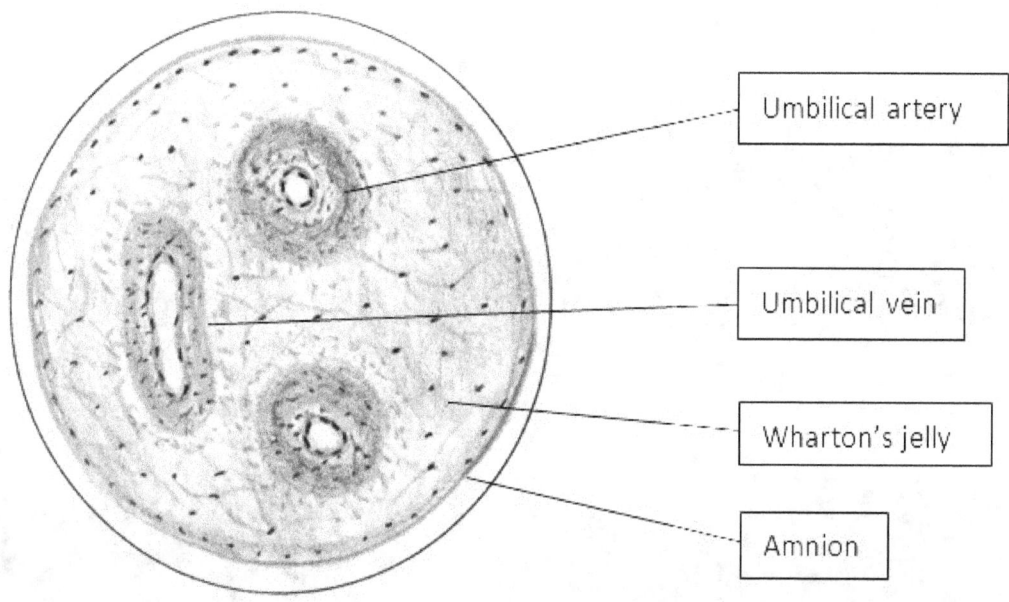

Cross Section of Umbilical Cord: 6